Move More, Your Life Depends On It:

Practical Tips to Add More Movement to Your Day

Amanda Sterczyk

The information in this book should not be used for diagnosis or treatment, or as a substitute for professional medical care. Before beginning any exercise program, consult your physician.

Excerpt from *Move Your DNA: Restore Your Health Through Natural Movement*, published by Propriometrics Press © 2014 Katy Bowman. Used with permission. All rights reserved.

Excerpt from "Rating of Perceived Exertion Scale," published by Productive Fitness © 2017. Used with permission. All rights reserved.

Excerpt from *Sitting Kills, Moving Heals: How Simple Everyday Movement Will Prevent Pain, Illness, and Early Death — and Exercise Alone Won't*, published by Quill Driver Books © 2011 Joan Vernikos. Used with permission. All rights reserved.

Excerpt from "Sedentary Behaviour Research Network (SBRN) — Terminology Consensus Project process and outcome," *International Journal of Behavioural Nutrition and Physical Activity* 14 © 2017 Mark S. Tremblay et al. Used with permission. All rights reserved.

Excerpt from "Why Seniors Fall," published by *Electronics Caregiver* © 2012 Robert Wood. Used with permission. All rights reserved.

Excerpt from *Fact Sheet on Physical Activity*, published by World Health Organization © 2014. Used with permission. All rights reserved.

Sterczyk, Amanda, author
Move More, Your Life Depends On It: Practical Tips to Add More Movement to Your Day / Amanda Sterczyk.

Includes bibliographical references.
Issued in print and electronic formats.

ISBN 9781720602415

1. Physical Fitness. 2. Sedentary Behaviour 3. Exercise & Fitness 4. Healthy Living

Editor: Kaarina Stiff
Cover: Dianna Little
Layout: Matthew Bin
Proofreading: Jennifer Rae-Brown
Author photo: Allison Mundle
Published by Amanda Sterczyk Fitness: AmandaSterczyk.com

To everyone who thinks
physical fitness is beyond their reach,
this book is dedicated to you.

Move more, feel better.

CONTENTS

INTRODUCTION

Physical inactivity is creating a global health crisis. Labour-saving devices and apps have reduced the need for us to get up and move, which is bad news for our health. Adding more movement to your day doesn't have to be complicated and it doesn't have to be time-consuming. If you're stuck and not sure what to do, just ask! That's what The Move More Institute™ is all about. With the guidance provided in this book, you can learn how to nudge yourself to be more active throughout the day, every day. But first, I want to recap why physical activity is so important.

Do you know the Rodin sculpture, "The Thinker"? If you've never seen this work of art, let me describe it to you. A very muscular, naked man sits with his elbow on his knee while his chin rests in his hand, and he appears deep in thought. He's a statue of a moment in time. That's how still and unmoving many people are for long periods of time. But let me tell you: You're not a statue, and you need to stop imitating one.

Being sedentary for too long impacts your entire body—your brain feels sluggish, your joints hurt, your muscles stiffen, and your mood turns generally gloomy. I think we can all agree that it's difficult to be a happy, productive person when you feel like that. Movement is key to happiness—even the famously happy Danes agree with me here.[1]

So what's your poison? Is it staying at your desk for hours on end? Or do you hunker down on the couch for an evening of binge-watching TV? Or both? Don't despair, you're not alone. For me, it's my hobbies. I like to read and knit. Both of these require me to sit still, and sometimes I forget to take a break and move around. That's why I decided to write this book. If I need help and nudges to get up and move, surely other people are in the same boat.

My business is physical activity. I'm a group fitness instructor and personal trainer. I have worked with men, women, and children aged three to 93 to help them improve balance, increase flexibility and strength, and understand the importance of daily physical activity. I have trained amateur athletes, weekend warriors, sedentary adults and seniors, children who sit still too much, individuals before and after surgical interventions, people with chronic medical conditions like diabetes (type 1 and type 2), Parkinson's disease, and multiple sclerosis, people who have just completed cancer treatments, and those recovering from broken bones or other injuries.

These people all have one thing in common: When they start to move their bodies, they feel better. I get people up and moving because if you move more, you will feel better. And yet, on occasion, I still don't move enough. Even when I was writing this book, I had to remind myself to stand up and move around every 30 to 40 minutes.

I hope that the information in this book will inspire you to add more movement to your day. I can't make your life less busy, but I can help make your life better by teaching you how to add natural movement—aka, non-exercise activity—to your busy life.

PART ONE:
THE PROBLEM

PHYSICAL INACTIVITY: WHAT'S THE PROBLEM?

Those who do not find time for exercise
will have to find time for illness.
— *Robert de Ferrers, 1st Earl of Derby, 1139*

Is Physical Inactivity a Global Health Problem?

The research is unequivocal: A sedentary lifestyle is hazardous to your health. Physical inactivity has been identified as the fourth leading risk factor for global mortality, behind high blood pressure, tobacco use, and high blood sugar.[2] A 2017 documentary on the rise of high cholesterol diagnoses provided further evidence of the phenomenon of death by lack of movement.[3] What's more, the World Health Organization attributes physical inactivity to 3.2 million premature deaths.[4]

Long periods of physical inactivity, whether you're stuck on a long flight or stuck in front of the TV, are harmful to your health. And active couch potatoes—people who meet the physical activity guidelines of 150 minutes of moderate to vigorous physical activity every week but who still spend long hours on the couch—are not immune from the ill effects of too much sitting. A study has confirmed that binge-watching TV is as bad as long-haul flights when it comes to increasing your risk of developing a potentially fatal blood clot.[5] The study's lead author recommended that we regularly get up and move around during leisure activities like watching TV. That type of movement is what I like to call "exercise snacks."

By the end of this book, I hope you'll see that my philosophy of healthy, active living includes these snacks of movement. Exercise AND non-exercise activity are vital to maintaining optimal health and preventing illnesses.

Are You a Prolonger or a Breaker?

Recent research has offered us a few ways to think about our activity levels.[6] A prolonger is someone who "accumulates sedentary time in extended continuous bouts." A breaker is someone who "accumulates sedentary time with frequent interruptions and in short bouts." We'll come back to these definitions in more detail in Part Three: The Action Plan.

These terms and their definitions come to us from the Sedentary Behaviour Research Network. Let's reflect on this network for a moment: Our society has become so sedentary for so long that researchers have had time to convene a worldwide research network to both study us and agree on common language about how little we move.[7] I used to work in health promotion research and let me tell you, nothing happens fast, especially a comprehensive project like this.

Is Sitting the New Smoking?

Do you have iPosture?[8] If you're hunched over your electronic device, your body position can negatively impact your self-esteem and mood, and a host of other things. (And the smaller the device, the bigger the hunch.)

The harm of our sedentary lifestyle has actually been years in the making. We've become a society of leisure-based, labour-saving, technological slugs, and it's killing us. Metabolic syndrome, type 2 diabetes, cardiovascular disease, and obesity are all on the rise.[9]

Sedentary living also increases our risk of developing some forms of cancer (colon, breast, endometrial).[10]

Unless you've been living under a rock for the past few years, you've likely heard the phrase "sitting is the new smoking." But please don't throw out your chairs just yet because sitting isn't the problem. Too much sitting is the problem—too many consecutive minutes and hours of sitting without regular breaks to stand up and move around.

What's wrong with sitting for too long? When we sit for too long, our bones are out of alignment and they stop doing their job. Our skeletons are designed to carry our body weight, but when the bones aren't aligned, the job falls instead to delicate connective tissue like tendons and ligaments. This can lead to soft tissue injuries, pain, and discomfort. In addition, when we don't use our bones to hold our bodies in motion, they become weak. And when the bones of our spine start to compress, we suffer from disc damage and loss of height.

The lack of movement from too much sitting also shortens our muscles (more on this in the next section on aging and physical inactivity), which means that they stop working together properly. Some muscles get tight, like our lower back and hips, while others get weak and overstretched, like our glutes and abs. This muscular imbalance can cause back pain because our muscles can't hold our bones in proper alignment.

Further up the body, our shoulders rotate, our head hunches forward, and our upper spine looks more like a T than a natural C curve. This gives us a sore neck, shoulders, and upper back, and makes it difficult to sit up straight. In turn, this imbalance of muscles—some tight, some weak, none functioning optimally—likewise impacts the range of motion in our joints, which translates to diminished balance and a heightened risk of falling.

Worried yet? That's not all. When our muscles don't function optimally, they stop helping our circulatory system pump blood to every nook and cranny in our bodies, reducing circulation. As a result, blood can pool in the feet and ankles because our muscles are not helping to pump that blood back up our bodies. Think swollen ankles, varicose veins, and blood clots.[11]

We'll practice a breathing exercise together later on because I want you to see that sitting causes our internal organs to lose real estate in our torso. When our organs are compressed, breathing and digestion become more difficult. And when our circulation has been downsized by lack of movement, our brain doesn't get enough oxygen and fresh blood. That's why we feel fuzzy and may have difficulty concentrating.

How do you feel when you sit too long? Can you relate to any or all of these physical effects of too much sitting? This is not a judgement of your level of physical inactivity, but rather a summary of the toll too much sitting takes on your body. And it also happens to my body when I sit too long. Now before you tell me we're just getting older, let me stop you right there.

Are You Aging or Just Physically Inactive?

Researcher and professor Robert Wood is featured in a YouTube video called "Why Seniors Fall." In it, he reported that half of the problems originally associated with aging are, in fact, the direct result of physical inactivity.[12] According to Professor Wood, "the person that has not been active has the most to gain by becoming active." I totally agree with Wood's assessment, which is why I recommend that people start with small snacks of activity. A little movement goes a long way. Let's examine what happens to our bodies when we're physically inactive and see how the effects can sometimes be misconstrued as aging.

When you stand up, how long does it take you to go from sitting to standing? Do you feel stiffness in certain joints as you get up? Those moving parts, aka your joints, are seizing up from lack of lubrication. It's like glue drying: The moisture in your muscles and joints disappears. When you are stiff, you move more slowly until you can get your joints and muscles lubricated by moving. Then, you can increase the speed of your movements. Here's how it works.

Your circulatory system relies on your muscular system to move blood and oxygen to all the cells in your body. When you stop moving parts of your body for extended periods of time, cells dry up and die. It starts with muscle atrophy; that is, the cells in your muscles shrink from non-use.[13] Your muscles shorten and pull the bones on either side of your joints closer together. Your muscles also become inflexible, which negatively impacts how much you can move—this is called the range of motion of your joints. That's why physically inactive individuals have a rounded back and stooped posture, not to mention a stiff and awkward gait that makes them appear older than they are.[14]

Why do we consider stiff and slow movements to be a sign of aging? Because older adults who are less active behave and move the same way. When I work with sedentary office workers in their 40s and 50s, they have the same physical issues as individuals in their 70s and 80s. When they get up and try to move around, these younger adults look older than they are.

Kind of scary, don't you think? Lack of physical movement is prematurely aging our society. So what's the solution? Move more. It's that simple.

Is "Labour-Saving" Killing Us?

How did this life of leisure entrap us in bodies that are now failing us? It was a gradual process throughout the twentieth century to our current times. The industrial revolution and technological revolution have given us many labour-saving devices. From dishwashers and garage door openers to smartphones and online shopping, researchers have tracked an increase in obesity that correlates directly with an increase in the acquisition of labour-saving devices.[15]

We have adopted a new lifestyle, one that entails less movement—under-moving, if you will—and it's not a healthy option. Biomechanist Katy Bowman said it well: "The frequent consumption of varied movement is what drives essential physiological processes. Movement is not as optional as we have led ourselves to believe. Just as lack of food (or, heaven forbid, oxygen) leads to a multitude of biological signals and physiological outcomes, people are living in their body-houses surrounded by screaming alarms in the form of pain, illness, and disease, and they are unaware of the source of the problem. You have been doing the movement equivalent of under-eating and under-breathing, which is having an impact on your whole body, right down to the cellular level."[16]

I like the term under-moving, because it has no emotional linkage to terms like "exercise" or "physical activity." Moving is what we do, what we NEED to do, every single day of our lives. And if you think about it, our brains are hard-wired to move. In fact, if you believe neuroscientist Daniel Wolpert, movement is the real reason for brains.[17]

And this under-moving can actually impact your breathing.

Do You Breathe Enough?

From weak muscles and stiff joints to sluggish brains and underperforming internal organs, a seated and slumped posture hurts your entire body. Try this simple breathing exercise.

If you're not already sitting, I want you to sit down and slump forward—the way you typically sit when you are hunched over your favourite electronic device—and then take a deep breath. Go ahead, do it.

How did it go? I'm guessing you couldn't fill your lungs completely. Now, try it again; but first, I want you to sit up straight, lower your shoulders down your back, and imagine that someone is pulling the top of your head toward the ceiling. Now give that a try.

Did it feel better? You were probably able to get more air into your lungs.

Next, stand up and repeat the breathing exercise. I'm sure you will agree that it was even easier to fill your lungs with air. Finally, I would like you to slowly walk around and again repeat the deep breathing task. Even better? You're welcome. Think about how much more oxygen is getting to every cell in your body now.

When I have people do this breathing exercise during my workshops, they are usually frustrated during the first try. But with each successive change, they smile more. They can see and feel for themselves how much better they feel when they sit up, get up, and walk around. Here's what one workshop participant told me via email.

"I just came home and my daughter was working at her computer. I told her to straighten her back and she said, 'WOW, I can breathe so much better!!!'"

Have You Tried a Standing Desk?

Too much sitting is bad for your health; you've now heard this message loud and clear. Unfortunately, you haven't received the follow-up memo: Too much stationary standing is equally bad for your health. Switching to a standing desk or a sit-to-stand desk is not the solution; you're just replacing one sedentary activity with another.[18]

One of my clients came to class one day complaining of a sore lower back. She told me this when I asked my standard start-of-class question, "Has anything changed in your body since the last time we saw each other?" Over the course of the class, she further revealed that her office switched from seated desks to standing desks. She told me that she was standing all day long because the office chairs had been removed from all the cubicles.

As I mentioned earlier, sitting in and of itself isn't the problem. Rather, it's too much sitting with no breaks to stand up and move. But too much standing without up and down movement is also a problem. And let's face it, sometimes we need to sit. Whether it's whilst driving or travelling by airplane (I'd like to see you ignore the "fasten seatbelt" sign during turbulence and see how long that lasts) or at a wedding.

What About When You Need to Sit?

By now, I hope you understand my stance on chairs and sitting. Sometimes we need to sit. Too much standing can also be problematic. Let me tell you a story to illustrate my point.

Many years ago, my then-boyfriend was invited to a wedding. Even though I had never met the bride (his friend) or anyone else involved in the nuptials, I was his "plus one." It was late August, and the heat was sweltering. We entered the church and gasped at the temperature inside. With no air conditioning and no windows to enjoy a breeze, it actually felt hotter in the church than outside.

The ceremony began and the officiant asked us to rise. What he forgot to do was indicate when we could sit down again. Being polite and attentive sheep, the entire congregation remained on its feet. I briefly noticed how dizzy I was becoming and then I just drifted toward the floor. Apparently, my one and only fainting episode was very graceful; bystanders remarked that I just "floated downwards."

I regained consciousness while four very large soldiers (it was a military wedding) were carrying me out of the church. Later, at the reception, I met the bride and groom for the first time. The bride said to me, "Oh, you're the one who took everyone's attention away from me on my big day." I think she was only half-joking. Nevertheless, this wedding was clearly a time when sitting would have been preferable to standing. The officiant even apologized for not instructing us to sit down.

And we mustn't forget about drummers. Their job requires them to sit, but they are anything but physically inactive. Watch a drum solo happen and you'll see how a drummer uses every muscle in their body. I can attest to the physical demands of playing the drums: A few years ago, I spent time learning to play. My body was anything but sedentary whilst seated at the drum kit.

Amanda: How Will You Sit Still to Write a Book?

One of my clients astutely observed that I would have difficulty sitting still to write. It takes A LOT of time to write a book, and sitting for long periods of time has been shown to be detrimental to everyone's health — mine included. But the content of my book wouldn't make sense if I couldn't even apply it to my own life!

So what did I do? I modified my work area to meet my needs. I wrote this book primarily on my laptop, and I regularly shifted locations and altered the height of my computer. I created a standing desk by stacking books on my kitchen counter and putting my laptop on top. Sometimes, I sat on the living room floor with my laptop on the coffee table or on my lap. Same goes for writing in bed—a pillow makes a nice laptop desk on my extended legs.

Writer's block was my cue to get up and move. If I was stuck on a particular section, I knew I needed to take a break from sitting still. Moving around helped me gather my thoughts and refresh my brain in the process. I emptied the dishwasher, played with our cat, puttered around the house, and went for walks. And if the weather was dreadful outside, I just paced around the house.

When I was out and about, I kept a pen and notepad in the car, in case inspiration struck. My social media followers had suggestions too, such as using the Notepad feature on my smartphone and setting up the "dictate to text" option on my smartphone. Both are great ideas that demonstrate a key premise of my work: an active lifestyle and modern conveniences do not need to be mutually exclusive. Although I've outlined the problems that labour-saving apps and devices have created, they can also offer us solutions too.

We've covered the problem of physical inactivity in this introductory chapter; now, let's turn our attention to physical activity.

But first, it's time for a break! You've been sitting long enough; time to get up and move. Don't worry, I'm not going anywhere. I'll be right here, waiting for you. Now go move your beautiful body!

PHYSICAL ACTIVITY:
HOW MUCH IS ENOUGH?

*Lack of activity destroys the good condition of every
human being, while movement and methodical
physical exercise save it and preserve it.*
— *Plato*

How Much Do Canadians Move Every Day?

Our bodies were designed to move, but how much do
most Canadians actually move every day? Not
enough, according to healthcare experts. And it's
costing us as a nation to the tune of 3.7 per cent of
overall health-care spending.[19]

The World Health Organization defines physical
activity as "any bodily movement produced by
skeletal muscles that requires energy expenditure."[20] I
don't see anything in that definition that mentions
sweating, special clothing, "feeling the burn," or

expensive gym memberships. What it does tell us is that movement—any movement—is physical activity. You need to move your muscles, or you will lose them. It's not rocket science, people!

Increasing the physical activity of Canadians would save lives—in excess of 6,600 premature deaths, or 2.4 per cent of the national population over a 25-year period. What's more, as a country that provides universal health care to its citizens, national healthcare costs and chronic conditions would decline with a modest increase in daily physical activity. We're talking thousands of fewer cases of cancer (31,000), type 2 diabetes (120,000), heart disease (170,000), and hypertension (222,000).[21]

Regular movement—loading your muscles and bones by working against gravity and then walking away from your desk—is what your body needs. Statistics Canada crunched the numbers and reported that you'll have a lower risk of premature death if you stand or walk around regularly, as opposed to staying seated for most of the day.[22]

So, how much should we move as Canadians? I'm glad you asked. Let's have a look.

How Much Should Canadians Move Every Day?

According to the Canadian Physical Activity Guidelines, adults need 150 minutes of moderate- to vigorous-intensity physical activity per week to maintain optimal health.[23] In the "moderate" category, examples include brisk walking and bike riding, whilst in the "vigorous" category, jogging and cross-country skiing are listed.

So, why exercise? It improves your fitness, strength, and mental health (morale and self-esteem), and it reduces your risk of premature death, heart disease, stroke, high blood pressure, certain types of cancer, type 2 diabetes, osteoporosis, and obesity.[24]

These are the minimum guidelines for physical activity. However, Statistics Canada data indicates that only 15 per cent of adult Canadians meet these minimum requirements.[25] Broken down to a daily level, the minimum exercise requirements—which were measured with accelerometers—equate to 21.42 minutes of daily exercise.

What are Canadian adults doing with their time when they are not exercising? They're being mostly sedentary, that's what—over 9.5 hours per day, which accounts for 69 per cent of their waking hours.[26] And, as we saw earlier, too much sedentary behaviour is creating a global health-care crisis.

Even if you meet the recommended physical activity guidelines, sedentary behaviour in the remaining hours of your day is still detrimental to your health.[27] Those remaining hours are the focus of this book. I will help you add non-exercise activity in common sense ways. Consistent with my original goal when I first created The Move More Institute™, I will share easy to implement and low-cost or free options. Let's go.

Can't You See My Bad Back Won't Let Me Exercise?

Ever heard someone say, "I have a bad back, so I can't exercise this week." Perhaps you've even said it yourself. But what exactly does it mean to have a bad back? Having a bad back implies you can't use it, and yet you use it every single day of your life, every time you move. Did you know that low back pain is the number two cause of work absenteeism?[28] And guess what? You're not alone in experiencing a bout of back pain during your lifetime.[29]

What causes low back pain? Some of the physical causes include lack of fitness, prolonged sitting, lifting heavy objects, operating motor vehicles, and having a history of smoking cigarettes. Our mostly sedentary lifestyle increases the risk of having a back pain attack. Think about it—you spend many of your waking hours seated, in a forward hunch. When you do get up, everything feels stiff and your posture is negatively impacted because you don't want to straighten up.

Here's the thing, stiffness begets stiffness. The less you move, the weaker and stiffer your muscles and joints become, and the harder it becomes to move easily and fluidly. So you move even less. What's a person with low back pain to do? Keep moving. Motion is lotion, after all, and the movement associated with your activities of daily living will slowly help to unlock the area of pain.[30]

That doesn't mean you should go run a marathon; be sensible about the intensity of your activity. A more recent study on treatments for low back pain advocates that practitioners should encourage patients to get out of bed and move. They are not advocating for a specific form of exercise, they are saying that their patients with low back pain should keep moving.[31]

When I'm working on something that excites me—like when I was writing this book—it can become all-consuming. It happened to me one lovely summer day a few years ago. I was evolving my business and updating my website. Before I knew it, I had been hunched over my laptop for over two hours, and I could feel the effects of that inactivity in my entire body. I decided to go for a walk to work out the kinks and think about next steps for my business, as well as run a few errands in the neighbourhood.

As I started down the sidewalk near our house, pain shot through my feet. As I mentioned, everything in my body had tightened up. Many times, I have had clients tell me they are too stiff to come to class or follow through with their training appointments. But I know first-hand that stiffness will go away with movement—that's why we always begin class and training sessions with a gentle warm-up. It gets the blood flowing and the engine humming before the more challenging work begins.

On that day, I slowed down my usual brisk pace and started breathing more deeply. The gentler speed combined with deep breathing was my warm-up before a brisk walk. I needed to keep moving to work out the kinks, but I needed to do it in a sensible way. And two blocks later, my body felt so much better and I was able to pick up the pace.

What Did You Do on Vacation?

Maybe you've heard this one before, too. A client goes to see their physiotherapist after returning from a vacation and says, "I'm healed! Must have been the sea air."

The therapist responds, "That's great! What did you do on vacation?"

"I walked around [insert exotic location here] day in and day out for a week."

"I see. And were you sitting at a desk for eight hours?"

"No, I was on vacation."

"Were you sitting on the couch binge-watching Netflix in the evening?"

"No, I was watching the local nightlife as I walked around."

"So, basically, your vacation involved leaving your sedentary habits at home and moving your body?"

"Yes, I guess you're right."

"Please try to incorporate some of your vacation habits back into your daily life. A little movement goes a long way, and it will definitely help you maintain good health and reduce the risk of re-injury."

A version of this anecdote was relayed to me by a physiotherapy colleague, who told me he hears stories like this quite often.[32] We humans sometimes work against our own best interests. Intellectually, we know that our bodies need to get up and move more to function optimally. And yet, we regularly stay seated and motionless for hours on end.

How Do You Accumulate Physical Activity?

Ready for some good news? The activity our bodies crave and need can happen in minuscule increments. Indeed, a study in the *Journal of the American Heart Association* reported that physical activity that was accumulated in sporadic bouts throughout the day still reduced the risk of early death.[33] The total amount of daily physical activity is more important than how you accumulate that activity.

What are your health or fitness goals? Disease prevention or injury prevention? Enjoyment of life? If you fall into one of these categories, there really is no need to go all out at the gym. For many people, their unspoken goals of fitness are basic to existence — prevent premature death and live life fully and pain-free. If you fall into this group, don't despair about people who may have more specific or rigorous fitness goals. You can focus instead on accumulating small, sporadic bouts of movement throughout your day. Every little bit counts toward your total physical activity: walking to the store, taking the stairs, or getting up from your desk and pacing during a conference call. As I mentioned before when describing my mission with The Move More Institute™, I call them "snacks of exercise." And these snacks don't require fancy workout clothes or special equipment, or the need to shower before continuing your day. Every little bit of movement matters. Just ask actress Eva Marie Saint.

"Did you know I'm older than the Oscars? Just keep moving."[34] Just. Keep. Moving. Those were the words Saint uttered at the 2017 Oscars. She was pondering the fact that the awards show was celebrating 90 years, and she was older at 93. And she looked fantastic, standing proudly, displaying every inch of her 5'4" frame—not stooped over and shuffling like many others later in their lives.

And she's right, you know. There is no secret elixir for aging well. You just have to keep moving. No fancy equipment or expensive gym membership required!

You know the drill: Time for a break! You've been sitting long enough; time to get up and move. Don't worry, I'm not going anywhere. I'll be right here, waiting for you. Now go move your beautiful body!

FROM NEAT™ TO ELITE: THE CONTINUUM OF PHYSICAL ACTIVITY

If we could give every individual the right
amount of nourishment and exercise, not too
little and not too much, we would have found
the safest way to health.
— *Hippocrates*

Why Do We Need to Move?

Every exercise is movement, but not every movement is exercise. And that's okay, because physical activity lies on a continuum, it's not an all-or-nothing endeavour. Just because you can't make it to the gym doesn't mean you can't be active. Rethink your activities: Go for a walk, play with your kids or grandkids, clean the house, or do some gardening. These are small steps that can lead to big change.

More and more research is validating my philosophy of activity. Whilst editing this book, yet another study was published about the importance of light physical activity to maintaining health and preventing premature death.[35]

Do you ever wonder why your brain feels cloudy when you've been immobile for a long period of time? As we discussed in the last chapter, motion is lotion, not just for your muscles and joints, but also for your brain. Your circulatory system relies on your muscular system to move blood and oxygen to all the cells in your body, including your brain.[36]

We were designed to be perpetual motion machines: If we stop moving, we stop working. Bottom line, we need movement—for our bodies, so our muscles don't atrophy, and for our brains, so they can function properly. But please do not interpret our need for movement as a call to "crush it" every time. I'm not joking here—some misguided souls assume every ounce of movement, not just the exercise bits— should involve maximal exertion. They've told me as much. Here is what happened.

I created a five-day movement challenge called "Get off your butt!" to help people whose jobs keep them sedentary for most of the day. The goal of the challenge was to add "snacks" of movement to their busy lives. The one-minute videos gave them quick and easy ideas to get them moving.[37] Participants also received a check-in email at the end of each day, to see how they did with the daily challenge.

One response I received from a participant was especially telling: "Not killing it but chugging along." Never did I ever instruct participants to "go all out" or "kill it" during these movement challenges. The premise behind the course was to add non-exercise activity to the workday. You know, stand up and reach your arms above your head. Repeat. Simple, sweat-free activities that get your blood moving and your muscles working.

Another participant shared the challenges with her colleagues. At the end of the week, she reported, "I think modifications to the exercises would be great for those of varying fitness levels. I found [for] my less active colleagues it was enough, but for myself and one other colleague, we needed more of a physical challenge."

I found it interesting that they interpreted the movement challenges as "exercises" that required varying degrees of intensity based on fitness level. This wasn't at all how I described the challenge, or my intention for it. It was all about non-exercise activity. With that in mind, let's take a moment to look more closely at the concept of non-exercise activity because it's really NEAT™.

What Is NEAT™?

NEAT™ refers to Non-Exercise Activity Thermogenesis—the way our bodies expend energy that is not by eating, sleeping, or working out.[38] These small, brief muscular movements are just as important as that gym workout in burning calories. You need both exercise and non-exercise activity in your life, but it's that non-exercise activity that we have lost in our daily lives.[39] That movement has been replaced by appliances and apps—labour-saving devices that have robbed our bodies of the physical activity, or labour, that we used to do on a daily basis before the technological revolution made movement almost obsolete.

NEAT™ is different than your workout at the gym because it relates to moving about in daily life.[40] Here's a comprehensive list of NEAT™ summarized by former NASA researcher Dr. Joan Vernikos, with an emphasis on changing position: "standing, lying, sitting down, bending over to pick something up, squatting, stretching upward to take something off a shelf, getting dressed and undressed, playing a musical instrument, stirring a pot, crossing and uncrossing one's legs, waving your hands while talking, and fidgeting."[41]

Our sedentary habits have erased these small movements from our repertoire. Even if you do a daily one-hour workout, you still need to keep your body moving in other ways throughout the day. If not, you're an active couch potato.[42] While active couch potatoes are better off than their sedentary counterparts, as measured by how many calories they've burned, they are actually worse off in the calorie-burning department than individuals who eschew the gym but move more throughout the day.[43]

Research suggests that light physical activity like NEAT™ is as beneficial to older adults and previously sedentary individuals as more vigorous exercise is for younger and more physically fit Canadians.[44] Our grandparents' generation didn't need fancy gym equipment or flashy workout gear. Their lives required more movement than our current way of living. There were no labour-saving devices like garage door openers, TV remotes, and online shopping. They didn't outsource physically demanding tasks like housework and snow shovelling. They just moved—a lot.

"Nein! Das ist mein Essen!"[45] yelled my husband's Oma when I tried to carry her groceries. It was the late 1990s and we were visiting Oma in Berlin, as she got ready for her 80th birthday. True to

German tradition, she was hosting her own birthday party.

Widowed a few years earlier, Oma lived alone in a one-bedroom apartment and walked to her local shops every day, as she had every day (except Sunday) for decades. Her tiny kitchen and even smaller fridge required daily visits to the grocery store. She was fiercely independent and proud that she could still carry her own groceries. That's what kept her strong and vital—she was still physically active on a daily basis.

Oma's small kitchen did not have a dishwasher, so after every meal she washed, dried, and put away the dishes. No dishes drip-drying on the counter, because she didn't have enough counter space to leave the dishes there. Like so many of her generation, the lack of labour-saving devices made her life more inconvenient than what younger generations enjoy. The upside? This inconvenience fuelled more non-exercise activity.

She also recycled almost everything, but the recycling bins were downstairs, outside her apartment building. So every day, after sorting metal, plastics, and paper, she ventured downstairs, walked outside, and reached up multiple times to empty her bags into the recycling bins. And there were no fancy workout clothes in Oma's closet—she did all of this in a skirt and sensible shoes.

There are so many ways that small movements and physical activity can be added to your daily life. Just ask the smart folks at ParticipACTION.

Is it Time for a Body Break?

I remember the ParticipACTION "Body Break" ads on TV from my childhood. This Canadian non-profit organization was founded in 1971 with a goal of decreasing Canadians' sedentary behaviour and encouraging them to move more.[46] Sound familiar at all?

Canada marked its 150th birthday in 2017. In the lead-up to Canada 150, ParticipACTION called on Canadians to submit entries for the Canada 150 Play List—150 ways for Canadians to move their bodies.[47] I submitted Essentrics® in the call for submissions. I have been teaching Essentrics® since 2010, when I switched careers and moved into the fitness industry.

Essentrics® and Classical Stretch™, the enormously popular TV version of the workout, engage your entire body in every workout. It's a full-body rebalancing program that focuses on maximum flexibility and strength for all 600+ muscles in your body. Men and women of all ages and ability levels, including elite athletes, do Essentrics®. Here was my rationale for submitting it to the Canada 150 Play List:

- Essentrics® is the only made-in-Canada fitness workout;
- There are trained instructors all across Canada;
- You can stream workouts online via Essentrics® TV;
- Creator Miranda Esmonde-White's TV show, Classical Stretch™, has been the #1 fitness show on PBS since 1999;
- You can purchase a multitude of DVDs for home use;[48] and,
- Esmonde-White has authored two best-selling books: *Aging Backwards*[49] and *Forever Painless*.[50]

That's a lot of ways for people across the country, and around the world, to practice Essentrics®. I was thrilled when Essentrics® was added as part of Activity 114 of 150: Fitness Activities.[51] The entire 150 Play List is awesome and, in my opinion, inspires movement and physical activity. From "no-equipment-required" activities like hide-and-seek, to equipment-laden activities like rowing, the list covers both ends of the continuum of physical activity, from easy to hard. And everything in between.

How Hard Are You Working?

Even though I'm not asking you to exercise, it's still useful to know how to measure your level of effort. The Rating of Perceived Exertion (RPE) is a scale used in the fitness world to subjectively measure how hard you're working during exercise; that is, how much you're exerting yourself. There are several scales available, but I prefer the 1–10 RPE scale that also includes the "talk test," produced and sold online by Productive Fitness.[52]

Here's a breakdown of the Exertion Scale and the corresponding zones:

Exertion Scale	Zone
1/2	Inactive
3/4	Health Improvement Zone
5/6	Fitness Zone
7/8	Performance Zone
9/10	High Performance Zone

A one-to-10 scale makes sense to most people and is something they can quickly comprehend. One represents low activity, like standing: minimal exertion and the ability to talk and breathe normally. Ten represents maximum intensity: the high performance zone, "severe" exertion and gasping for breath, like you're in a race that you're trying to win.

And, of course, every number from one to 10 represents an incremental increase in exertion, corresponding to a decrease in the ability to talk and breathe as you would whilst at rest. Makes sense, don't you think?

When I'm teaching classes or training people, I regularly reference the Rating of Perceived Exertion scale because I believe that different activities should be performed at different levels. Unless you're an elite athlete or a weekend warrior in competition, is there really a need to perform at 9/10? A rhetorical question, to which I would say, "No."

When you overlay the RPE scale with the concepts of NEAT™ and the continuum of physical activity described earlier in this chapter, I'm sure you would agree that most NEAT™-defined activities take place in the zones 1/2 and 3/4.

In my practice, I also emphasize the importance of activities that take place in zones 1/2 and 3/4 because those are the activities we have abandoned as a culture, like our Activities of Daily Living, which I will talk about next.

Can You Brush Your Own Hair?

After grad school, I worked in health promotion research, studying fall prevention among the elderly. It was through this work that I first learned about activities of daily living (ADL),[53] a term used in health care to determine a person's ability to care for themself. Some people don't like one of the mnemonics used to remember ADLs: DEATH— Dressing/bathing, Eating, Ambulating (walking), Toileting, Hygiene.[54] Personally, I like it. If you can't independently complete these basic ADLs, you're more likely to be knocking at death's door. These activities indicate how well you can function on your own.

There's also a second level of ADLs, called instrumental activities of daily living (IADLs). Their mnemonic is SHAFT: Shopping, Housekeeping, Accounting, Food preparation/meds, Telephone/transportation. Sounds like more movement that allows independence AND keeps your body moving. But I digress.

Let's return to the original list of ADLs. Can you put on a shirt unaided? Can you lift a fork to your mouth? Can you get in and out of bed? Can you sit down on the toilet and get up again unaided? Can you brush your own hair or teeth? All of these activities require motion, movement, and physical activity. Call it what you will—I call it using your body to take care of yourself.

We've pretty much covered the entire continuum of physical activity, except for the high performance or elite end of the spectrum, which deserves a few words too.

How Hard Does an Elite Athlete Work?

Patrick Smith is an elite triathlete. That means he excels at three sports: swimming, cycling, and running. He spends a lot of time training and competing. At this point in his life, it's his full-time job.[55]

Growing up, Patrick's life was focused around sports, and he began swimming competitively at the age of eight. He was also running at school, both track and cross-country, but since swimming was his main passion, the running served as cross-training and a way to stay in shape for swimming.

Nowadays, he's competing at the top level in his sport, with his eye on the 2024 Paris Olympics. His races cover a lot of distance both in the water and on land, and are classified as Sprint or Olympic distance:

Race Type	Sprint	Olympic
Swim Portion	750 metres	1,500 metres
Cycle Portion	20 kilometres	40 kilometres
Run Portion	5 kilometres	10 kilometres

As I said, Patrick's main focus in life is triathlon training and competition. He spends 18 to 24 hours training every week: 22 to 24 hours if he's in full training mode, and 18 hours if he's tapering his training in the 10-day lead-up to a competition. But in both cases, only a small fraction of that time is spent at the high-performance level. Here's how Patrick explains it: "You have to find a balance. You can train at a nine or 10 but you have to be able to come back the next week, the next month, and stay injury-free." That doesn't mean the remainder of his training time is spent at the performance level—that is, 7/8 on the RPE scale. In fact, the bulk of his training time is spent at the fitness level, 5/6 on the RPE scale:

	Training Week	Competition Week
5/6 – Fitness Level	11–13 hours	10–12 hours
7/8 – Performance Level	5–7 hours	2–4 hours
9/10 – High Performance Level	3–5 hours	3–5 hours

Even at the elite level, athletes are paying attention to the continuum of physical activity and adapting their training accordingly. They balance high intensity and lower intensity workouts on a daily basis; their "zero to 60" performance only kicks in at specific times. They pace themselves, and so should you.

You know the drill: Time for a break! You've been sitting long enough; time to get up and move. Don't worry, I'm not going anywhere. I'll be right here, waiting for you. Now go move your beautiful body!

PART TWO:
THE SOLUTION

INSIDE THE MOVE MORE INSTITUTE™

Exercise to stimulate, not to annihilate. The world
wasn't formed in a day, and neither were we.
Set small goals and build upon them.
— Lee Haney

Have You Heard the Tale of Two Clients?

Let me tell you a tale of two personal training clients.
One of my training clients ended our sessions because
of cost and scheduling. He was planning to join a gym
and work out on his own instead. After spending one
hour a week with him for two months or so, I set up
some training programs for him to complete on his
own. And, of course, I reminded him about the
importance of staying active every day, not just at the
gym once or twice a week. A few months later, he
emailed to thank me for all I'd done for him. Even
though he'd only been my client for a short while, he

told me I got him on the path to health and wellness. He said that thanks to me, he was living a better life.

At the same time, I had another client who was doing great during her workouts with me, but was more or less inactive during the rest of her waking hours. Although she thrived during our sessions, I could see that it wasn't impacting her life in the way she wanted. I always gave her "homework" — exercises for her to be doing on her own. But each time we met, she provided a multitude of excuses for why she hadn't done the work.

Reflecting on these two clients, I realized that I wanted to do more than just train people at a gym. I wanted to have a positive impact on their whole lives, so they could enjoy life. A weekly personal training session of one hour accounts for less than one per cent of a person's waking hours. I wanted to influence more of people's lives. I wanted them to get active and stay active every single day. If we only rely on that "less than one per cent" block of time to change your behaviour, how successful do you think you'll be? (Psst. Rhetorical question alert.)

The point is, a one-hour workout with a personal trainer is devoted to exercise, not behaviour change. Coaching for behaviour change is a key foundation of The Move More Institute™ because I want you to be more active when you're going through your daily life. You, or any of my clients for that matter, are already more active during personal training sessions and group fitness classes. I also want you to get moving during the other 99.992 per cent of your waking hours. That's the key to feeling better, enjoying life, and reducing your risk of premature death.

My new goal required a paradigm shift in how I approached my profession.

What Was My Paradigm Shift?

As I was developing The Move More Institute™, I realized that we need a paradigm shift to address our sedentary lifestyle. As a personal trainer and fitness instructor, my goal has always been to get people to exercise more: join a class, hire me to get them working out or to create a training plan for them, or bring me in to teach a lunchtime exercise class. You get the idea.

Yet, research shows that not only are Canadians not exercising enough, they're also not moving enough. And I had seen what happens when people try to go from "zero to 60" in a short amount of time. They get injured or they feel overwhelmed by working out so much after a period of physical inactivity. In other words, they do too much, too fast, and they burn out as a result.

I knew there had to be a better way to get people moving and keep them moving. I decided to delve into my education and training to research various behaviour change models, in the hopes of finding solutions that would stick. I wanted to show people that they have the power to make a positive change in their lives, and that they don't need to spend a ton of money on equipment or training to feel better. After all, the movement I was suggesting was simple yet NEAT™.

There is still no magic pill for exercise.[56] But NEAT™ is free and easy; it's different than a workout at the gym. You don't need fancy clothes, complicated equipment, or an expensive gym membership to add NEAT™ to your day.

Remember what NEAT™ is? It refers to Non-Exercise Activity Thermogenesis and it's the way our bodies expend energy that is not by eating, sleeping, or working out.[57] And these small, brief muscular movements often burn more energy than a gym workout. In practice, you need both exercise and non-exercise activity in your life. But I'm here to help you add the non-exercise activity back in your life.

Have You Ever Had a Radical Idea?

Here's a radical idea: I'm a fitness professional and I'm telling you not to exercise. Keep reading and I'll explain myself.

Here's what I want for you: Natural, non-exercise activity spread throughout your day. Every day. There have been dozens (and dozens) of articles written about "finding YOUR workout" because you're more likely to stick with an exercise or sport that you enjoy. If you hate that 6:00 a.m. boot camp and it's making your life miserable, don't do it! If "exercise" turns your stomach and you hate the thought of schlepping to the gym, don't do that either!

My comment about not exercising is only partly tongue-in-cheek. I would much rather you be active with non-exercise activity every day of your life, than forcing yourself to do a twice-weekly workout that makes you unhappy. That's why I created The Move More Institute™. Ideally, I would love for everyone to be physically active with both exercise and non-exercise activity. But as you saw earlier in the book, most Canadians aren't doing enough of either type of movement. And some researchers have proposed that fitness professionals recommend both exercise and non-exercise activity to their clients—an acknowledgement that exercise on its own is not enough to counteract the deleterious effects of too much sedentary behaviour.[58]

The Move More Institute™ promotes healthy, active living by adding more movement to individuals' daily lives. You know, the way we used to move as kids. Well, I can't speak for you and your childhood, but it's how I used to move as a child. For the moment, let's pretend our childhoods were similar whilst we reminisce.

Remember Your Childhood?

Remember the carefree summer days of your (my) childhood, when you would jump out of bed with enthusiasm, ready for whatever adventure presented itself? The world was full of possibility and so were you. You didn't think twice about hopping on your bike to race to your best friend's house. When you arrived, you kicked off your shoes and ran through the sprinkler until you were too hungry to continue. After a quick lunch, it was time to head to the park, until you were called home for dinner.

You didn't have to think about your posture, proper knee alignment when bending your legs, shoes to support your weak arches, or range of motion in your joints. You just did what came naturally and you moved—a lot.

How does your body feel these days? Do you still jump out of bed and run around in your bare feet? Likely not, as most adults report some form of muscular or joint pain. Even though our bodies have evolved to be physically active, many of us don't move enough during the day. Who knew that the industrial revolution would precipitate such a polar shift in our activity levels? As society has advanced, the technological changes have altered our lifestyles dramatically. More people spend most of their waking hours immobile, in a seated position. They are sitting during the morning and evening commutes, sitting at a desk, and slouching on the couch in the evenings while they binge-watch their favourite shows on demand.

What Is The Move More Institute™?

The Move More Institute™ is a 20th-century solution for a 21st century problem. My goal is to make your life a little less convenient so you have to add more movement to your day. I want you to do things that nudge you to do more activity, so that you have to move more without thinking about it. People used to HAVE to move more in their daily life, so they did.

My slogan is Move More, Feel Better. I like to think of NEAT™ as "pre-exercise." That is, eschewing the modern-day trappings of exercise for good old-fashioned movement.

My grandmother never had a pair of runners, let alone workout clothes. I only remember her wearing dresses; in fact, I don't think I ever saw her in a pair of pants. Yet, she was incredibly strong and healthy until she died. And my grandparents' house was not chock full of labour-saving devices or convenience set-ups.

They had a manual garage door that my grandmother would open, then get in the car, drive the car out of the garage, get out of the car, and close the garage door before getting back in the car to drive away. It was a heavy door, too. They only had one phone, which was on the wall in the kitchen—no quick "hello"s after reaching into your back pocket to answer the call. The TV did not have a remote control—you had to stand up and walk to the TV to change channels and mute commercials (and my grandfather hated commercials, so there was a lot of muting going on). Their vacuum cleaner was a beast, heavy and unmanoeuvrable, and my grandmother vacuumed almost every single day. In the kitchen, there were only basic appliances: no dishwasher, no electric mixer, no electric can opener. Food prep and clean-up happened by hand, many times throughout the day. Like I said, every single day.

I often suggest that people pretend they're living in the 1980s. Under the guise of #ThrowbackThursday I remind them that they used to walk down the hall to converse with a colleague. And remember going to the mall to buy a book or a bottle of shampoo? Instead of using a smartphone to shop online, why not head to a store and walk around while you peruse the offerings? When my daughter was younger, she used to call it "window buying." And I willingly took her window buying because it encouraged her to walk for pleasure.

But these non-exercise activities are no longer second nature for people. We need to re-educate ourselves on how to add activity to our lives and how easy it is to do. That's where psychology and behavioural science come in, topics I know well.

My background includes two social psychology degrees, almost 10 years working in health promotion research, and over nine years in the fitness industry. All of these fields rely on behaviour change to help people. And I have spent more than two years researching behaviour change as it specifically relates to movement, exercise, and physical activity. Now,

I'm not going to bore you with a lot of technical mumbo-jumbo (you're welcome). Instead, I will focus on the key behaviour change models that I have incorporated into The Move More Institute™.

First, I'll explain the models. Then the rest of this book will teach you how to add movement in specific ways, incorporating components of these behaviour change models.[59]

You know the drill: Time for a break! You've been sitting long enough; time to get up and move. Don't worry, I'm not going anywhere. I'll be right here, waiting for you. Now go move your beautiful body!

BEHAVIOUR CHANGE MODELS AND THE MOVE MORE INSTITUTE™

Walking is the best possible exercise.
Habituate yourself to walk very far.
— *Thomas Jefferson*

How Does the Power of Habit Impact Behaviour Change?

Before we jump into nudges, let's talk about behaviour change. It's a favourite topic of mine that I have studied extensively. Behaviour change is a popular topic in the fitness industry because personal trainers need to understand how to motivate people to change (that's kind of their job).

One of the biggest challenges when helping people change their behaviour is teaching them about the power of habit. A habit, or routine, is a behaviour that is so ingrained that you don't do it consciously.

Take a moment to think about what you do when you wake up in the morning. Let's examine my weekday morning routine as an example.

My alarm goes; I turn it off and get up. I put on my housecoat and go downstairs. First task is coffee: Grind the beans, fill the coffee pot with water, put a filter in the filter basket, put the coffee in the basket, pour the water into the coffeemaker, and hit the brew button. While the coffee brews, I feed the cat and the gerbils. (They may want to eat first thing in the morning, but I prefer to have my coffee first!)

I'm not focused too closely on my behaviour. I'm tired because I just woke up and haven't yet had coffee (duh). But also, I've done the same thing so many times that it's automatic. It's my morning routine. Wash. Rinse. Repeat.

So, what happens when my routine is switched up? One morning, the cat arrived in the kitchen early and started meowing for her food, very loudly, I might add. So loudly, in fact, I was worried she'd wake up the household. I'm a much happier person if my first coffee of the morning is consumed in peace, without children needing attention, chatting, or wanting some of my precious coffee. (Now that they're teenagers, it's a thing. They actually want coffee too. MY coffee. But I digress.)

I paused my regular morning routine and fed the cat immediately.[60] And when I got back to making coffee, I promptly poured the ground coffee into the filter basket BEFORE I placed a coffee filter in the basket. What a mess! I had to clean it up and start again. My morning routine was such a habit that I couldn't complete it properly when a wrench—or cat—was thrown into my system.

Behaviours that are habits fall into what is called the habit loop, where we don't realize on a conscious level what is cueing this behaviour and what reward we are seeking from it.[61] In the case of my morning routine, coffee is clearly my external reward. The underlying, or internal, reward is a bit of me-time as I ease into my day. Charles Duhigg eloquently identifies and describes the habit loop in his book, *The Power of Habit*. I recommend you read his book and visit his website if you want to delve further.[62]

Before you can change a behaviour, you need to understand the existing behaviour's habit loop. That means recognizing the unconscious triggers—the who, what, when, where, or why that set off the behaviour—and knowing the internal rewards for the behaviour. For the purpose of this book, we will not break down the habit loop; I have provided links to the habit expert for that. Instead, I want to work with you on creating external cues that you can practice in your daily life.[63] These cues, or nudges, will serve to get you moving more because they will change your habitual behaviour of remaining sedentary. Just like the cat cued a change in my morning habit of making coffee, although in that case, the behaviour change was not a desired one!

How Does a Baby Learn to Walk?

Have you ever watched a baby learning to walk? They take baby steps—after a few tentative steps, they fall, and they get up and try again. Babies don't know that learning a new behaviour is hard work. They just keep getting up and trying over. First it's a few steps with a fall, then it's walking, then running. It's a long process that begins with one step. I know that may sound corny, but it's a great analogy for behaviour change. Start small and keep at it.

Psychologist BJ Fogg coined the term "tiny habits" to capture the principle of baby steps for behaviour change.[64] Believe it or not, I first heard the term in a movie. The 1991 comedy *What About Bob?* starred Richard Dreyfus as a brilliant psychotherapist who had just published a book called Baby Steps. And Bill Murray was his accidental patient who quickly adopted the behaviour change model and was able to conquer his anxiety and obsessive-compulsive disorder.[65]

The overarching message with baby steps is that you shouldn't look at the big picture and what you're trying to achieve. You shouldn't look any further than the end of your nose. Take baby steps, one small step at a time. The concept of baby steps also reminds me of a great motherhood statement, "You can't boil the ocean." But you can take one tablespoon from the ocean and boil it. My goal with The Move More Institute™ is to get you up and moving using nudges and baby steps. Why? Because something is better than nothing and you'll be starting a journey that will benefit your entire body.

Baby steps.

What About WALL-E?

Have you seen the 2008 Pixar animated movie WALL-E? In it, the humans move around on floating beds with nary a glance at their "strolling" companions. The human bodies are shapeless and undefined, and they use a video monitor at the end of their noses to communicate with other humans who are within arm's reach. Basically, they have outsourced the job of their muscles to technology.

I always saw this view of humanity as a cautionary tale, a glimpse into where we are headed if we don't modify our sedentary lifestyle. Toward the end of the movie (spoiler alert, skip this section if you plan on watching it), the humans start to leave the moving beds. The first tentative steps they take on their own are reminiscent of a baby learning to walk. Indeed, they haven't used their muscles in so long, it's as if they're starting from scratch. But, like babies, they persevere and learn to walk again on their own two feet—the way we evolved to move.

What Is Nudge Theory?

My goal with The Move More Institute™ is to nudge people to be more active throughout the day. So, what exactly is a nudge? Thank you for asking!

A nudge is simply a way to draw your attention; for instance, putting something at eye level so you notice it. Nudge theory, popularized by behavioural economist Richard Thaler, involves creating small changes in the environment that are designed to change someone's behaviour.[66] These nudges should be inexpensive and easy to implement, such as leaving fresh fruit on the counter to encourage healthy food choices.

When someone wants to change a habit, nudges are often recommended. Want to exercise more? Leave those running shoes beside your bed, so you see them as soon as you wake up in the morning. In this way, "out of sight, out of mind" is the polar opposite of nudge theory. And with people's busy lives, if you're always putting your runners in the closet, how likely is it that you'll retrieve them to go for a run or a power walk? It's not very likely at all.

Nudges are not age-specific, either. One day as I was vacuuming, I asked my teenage son to move his muscle roller, which had taken up residence on the hallway floor outside his bedroom door. His response? "Forever or just while you vacuum? I like to leave it there so it reminds me to roll my muscles. If I don't see it, I forget to do it." Of course I told him he could return it to its nudge spot when the vacuuming was done. I know too well how easy it is to forget to do something when your reminder is out of sight.

After reading extensively on nudges and nudge theory, I started wondering how to add movement-based nudges to my clients' lives. Remember, nudges should be inexpensive (free is even better), easy to implement, and guide someone toward the behaviour you are trying to encourage. In my case, I recommend nudges to get you to sit less and move more. One of my favourite nudges is the simple sticky note, which I describe below. I hope that this section on solutions will help you think of your own novel nudges that will work better for you!

Can You Post Your Nudge?

Has this ever happened to you? You've got a deadline, so you hunker down to work but you just keep spinning your wheels. This has happened to me too. One day, I had a list and I was determined to complete everything on that list. At one point, I was feeling foggy-headed, so I thought about going for a walk to clear my head. But I didn't. I stayed working on my laptop instead. I wanted to cross everything off that list as soon as possible.

And do you know what happened? Nothing, that's what. I could not focus on my deliverables, which means I didn't meet my deadline.

It happens to the best of us—when life piles on more tasks, we tend to get overwhelmed and less productive. That night, as I was going to bed, I made a promise to myself: that I would set a reminder to get up and move. So, I wrote on a few sticky notes and placed them strategically around the house—on the edge of my computer screen, beside my water glass, on the back of the bathroom door (you know, for when you're sitting and contemplating life). They all had simple messages: Go for a walk; get up and move; stretch your arms.

Why does this work? When you are juggling lots of balls, it's tough to throw a new behaviour into the mix. Your brain just won't remember to do this new activity because you haven't yet created the neural pathways to make it a habit. That's where nudges help—they are visual cues that help move you toward the new behaviour. And when they work, you feel fantastic!

I received the following message from a friend one day: "Hi Amanda! I took your advice and went on a power walk at lunch! I had been working on month-end reports and needed to get my blood and heart pumping because I was getting sluggish!! I feel so alive again!! #keepmoving." Catherine had seen my social media post about needing to clear my brain and how I used sticky notes to nudge my desired behaviour. It inspired her to get up and move more, even when she was facing a deadline at work.

After the inaugural five-day movement challenge, which I will tell you about in the next chapter, one participant told me, "The sticky notes were an awesome idea that I will keep using in my daily life." It's a nudge that is inexpensive, easy to implement, and helps you adopt your new behaviour of moving more. That's what I'd call a win-win!

You know the drill: Time for a break! You've been sitting long enough; time to get up and move. Don't worry, I'm not going anywhere. I'll be right here, waiting for you. Now go move your beautiful body!

BREAKING DOWN YOUR BARRIERS TO MOVING MORE

Being busy does not always mean real work.
— Thomas Edison

How Do I Spend My Time?

Doing an audit of your day is a great way to get you thinking about physical activity. When you start to examine the specific activities you do each hour, you can see how much you move (or don't move). I created "activity clocks" to provide a visual depiction of a daily audit. Let's do one together.

Get a paper and pen, and draw two circles. Add lines to divide each circle into 12 equal sections— imagine a big pie being sliced up. Each circle represents 12 hours, so the two circles together represent a typical 24-hour day. Write the hours of the day around each circle to make them look like real clocks.

This process is about identifying what activities you do in each hour. Many of these activities last less than an hour, for example, eating breakfast. To most accurately represent how much time we spend on different things, I find it's easier to think about things in 30-minute increments. Now, fill in each segment to capture what you do. You can use symbols to differentiate various activities. For example, use * for exercise, ^ for eating, + for screen time—you get the idea. Or, if you prefer, you can use different coloured pens or pencils to represent different activities.

Keep the following in mind as you complete your clocks:

- The average adult sleeps from seven to nine hours.
- Eating should include food prep time. Food prep is non-exercise activity, and eating is a way we expend energy. So, although you're sitting while you eat, that's a perfect example of when sitting is acceptable (and even desirable).
- Screen time includes working on a computer, watching TV, or using a smartphone.
- Commuting should distinguish between passive commuting (car or bus or train) and active commuting (walking or running or

bicycling); this includes both commuting for work and running errands or driving yourself and others to activities.

- Household duties include housekeeping, caring for loved ones or pets, or anything else on the home front that gets you moving.
- Exercise should be listed separately from non-exercise activity and then included in the total for movement.
- Leisure activities include hobbies that require little or no physical activity and are mostly sedentary (e.g., reading, writing, knitting, sewing).

Now, add the total time for passive commuting, working, screen time, and leisure activity. This is your total sedentary time: the portion of your life when you're sitting too much and the one you have identified as needing to change.

Once you have done a visual audit of your typical day, I'm hoping you'll find it easier to spot opportunities to add small bits of movement to your day. Remember, adding NEAT™ movements is about nuggets of activity. No matter what your results show, don't feel badly about your level of sedentary behaviour. The activity clocks are meant to help you visualize how you can add movement, not shame you because you're sedentary.

Am I "Too Busy"?

Let's be clear: I am not judging your activity level. Everyone has commitments and people who rely on them. And you're not alone. Be it school, a new job, marriage, a new home, or children, life gets in the way of even the best intentions. Your plate is full and when there's no room left on the plate, something has to give. And often, exercise slides off the plate first.[67]

Having said that, "busy" should not be a badge of honour. We all get the same 24 hours every day. In reality, you're doing yourself (and those who rely on you) a disservice when you forgo your own needs. You will feel better and perform better—regardless of what you need to be doing—if you move more.[68]

One reason that is true is that regular movement helps prevent injury and illness. Because (rhetorical question alert) how will you get everything done if you fall ill or injure yourself? Remember all those people relying on you at home and work? You're no good to any of them if you fall apart.

The activity clocks provide a visual audit of your day to help you figure out what's making you so busy. They will show you how much of your typical day is spent on activities that are mostly sedentary.

Breaking down your day allows you to understand where you can add those nuggets of movement—or snacks of exercise—to get you moving more. One client who used the activity clocks to audit her day discovered that after driving her daughter to hockey practice, she usually sat in the stands for the next hour. She decided, instead of sitting for an hour, to walk around inside the arena on cold days, and walk outside on warmer days. She told me that their drive home after practice is now less stressful because she feels better and she's able to cope better with the rush-hour traffic.

Now that we've examined your entire day, let's break down your desk set-up and see how you can make some small changes to increase your movement factor while you're at your desk. We will do this using the inconvenience set-up rating.

What Is the Inconvenience Set-Up Rating?

The inconvenience set-up rating is a way to assess your workspace. When you're sitting at your desk, is everything within easy reach? This "convenience set-up" is part of the problem when it comes to sedentary behaviour. If you never have to get up to fetch your water, answer the phone, or pick up a printout, inactivity becomes the norm.

Take a look at your desk and count how many of your everyday items are within arm's reach. More items within easy reach means a lower inconvenience set-up rating. On a scale from one to 10, one is very convenient and 10 is inconvenient. In this case, convenience is a bad thing, because a very convenient desk set-up negatively impacts your movement.

There are no right or wrong answers here, we're just trying to assess your current set-up and determine how to improve it. If you shift things to be just a little bit more inconvenient, it will nudge you to move more.

This assessment of your space has two parts. First, rate your current inconvenience set-up from one to 10. If you rate your space at the low end of the scale, consider implementing more than one of the following suggestions as you modify your workspace. That's the second part of the assessment.

- At your desk, how can you reduce your convenience set-up?
- Is your water bottle out of reach, up high if possible?
- Is your phone just far enough away so you have to stand up to answer it?
- Are your documents within easy reach, or are you getting up and walking around your desk to retrieve them?

- Is your printer on the edge of your desk or do you send print jobs to a device that is farther away?

- If you have a home office, are you reaching across your desk to print or photocopy documents? Or do you take advantage of being out of your chair to walk a little further? I call this manoeuvre "taking the long cut": Do a lap of your entire home to reach the printer or photocopier on your desk, then retrace your steps to "return" to your office.

This last point of "taking the long cut" extends your inconvenience set-up beyond your immediate workspace. So, for example, consider a washroom break that involves taking the stairs and going to another floor, or simply walking around the perimeter of your home before you arrive at the washroom outside your home office.

Isn't There an App for That?

I bet some of you are thinking, "There's an app for that, there's a device for that." Be it an app for your smartphone or smart watch, or a stand-alone device like a pedometer or other fitness tracker that you clip to your waistband, there are many products on the market geared to getting and keeping you active. If you're using one or more of these tools and they're helping you, fantastic! I want you to move more every day, regardless of what gets your activity level up.

However, I suspect you're not, and that's why you bought this book. Everyone is wired differently and not everyone is motivated by apps or so-called smart devices, and fitness trackers don't always work the way you intended.

Just as it's possible to under-exercise, it's also possible to over-exercise. If you are using a fitness tracker that encourages addictive behaviour, too much exercise may become a problem for you. It did for Professor Zoë Chance from the Yale School of Management.[69] Take a few minutes to watch her story of the pedometer that became her addiction. Her TEDx Talk is about 16 minutes long, but I'm focusing on the first half of the video.

For those of you who want the condensed version of Chance's talk, here it is. (If you want to watch the video first, go ahead and check back with us when you're done.) Chance describes how purchasing a pedometer negatively impacted her life. While most people using pedometers aim for 10,000 steps per day, Chance was logging 24,000 steps per day. You see, her pedometer kept sending her challenges to complete, including consecutive challenges in the middle of the night that had her climbing 2,000 steps up and down in her basement for points—at 2:00 a.m.

I'm sure many of you can relate to the thrill of accomplishing the milestones set by her pedometer. But when it is impacting your overall health and judgement—her sore neck, her sister's choice to walk miles alone in the middle of the night, checking the pedometer results every five minutes—perhaps the costs outweigh the benefits of more movement and activity.

The lesson here is that, on their own, pedometers and other fitness trackers can sometimes give you a skewed interpretation of your physical activity level. You shouldn't rely solely on that data to gauge your physical activity.[70] These tools fail to capture the quality of your exercise:

- How vigorously are you walking?
- Is the surface flat or steep?
- How long is it taking you to walk those steps?

Addiction and over-reliance on technology are two key downsides to using fitness trackers.[71] But in my mind, they are pretty big red flags. Not to mention the detachment from actually listening to your body. If you use a fitness tracker and you're able to do it responsibly, more power to you. But for the rest of us, let's agree to pay more attention to warning signs in our bodies that tell us to get up and move more.

Want to Hear My Fitness Tracker Story?

My experience with a fitness tracker was somewhat different. As a fitness instructor, I teach a unique dynamic stretching program called Essentrics®. In 2014, I was teaching A LOT of Essentrics®—about 15 weekly sessions, including group classes and private sessions, in eight different locations. I was teaching schoolchildren, athletes, and adults of all ages. I'm sure you'll agree that I was getting a lot of exercise—much more than the recommended 150 minutes a week.

Around the same time, I decided to buy a fitness tracker. Don't ask me why, I can't recall. Even though my body knew it was working hard with all that Essentrics®, perhaps my brain needed data to validate my activity level.

For two weeks, I wore the fitness tracker every waking hour. I put it on my bedside table, and I slipped it onto my pyjama bottoms as I got out of bed. The tracker recorded a lot of steps in the morning and evening, which is no surprise to any mom with school-age children. Interestingly, though, the tracker did not pick up any "movement"—displayed as number of steps—when I was teaching Essentrics®. And yet, I was exercising a lot.

I decided to ditch the fitness tracker and listen to my body. I was moving and I was exercising, regardless of what the fitness tracker said about my activity level. Why did I need to rely on technology to tell me if I needed to move? Rhetorical question, friends. I much prefer to rely on my body and its internal fitness tracker to tell me to get up and move.

Can Technology and an Active Lifestyle Co-Exist?

Sometimes, technology can be our friend AND help our bodies. Take headphones or earphones, for example. Some people think too many younger adults are disengaging by moving through life with headphones or earphones always connected to their auditory channels. That may be true for some individuals, and I'll admit that I sometimes use music to drown out the outside world, but not always.

One morning, I was scheduled to be on a video conference call at my desk, but my teenage son was home from school due to illness. He wanted to sleep, so I changed my video conference to a regular phone call. Then I popped in my earphones, put on my sunglasses, and headed out for a walk. For an hour, I walked around the neighbourhood, attending to the business at hand and getting some fresh air and exercise in the process. I accomplished just as much as I would have inside, and I felt great. Plus, I got that much-needed Vitamin D boost that so many of us lack in the winter months. I'd say it was a win-win. And it's a clear example of when an active lifestyle and modern conveniences need not be mutually exclusive.

Video-streaming services like Netflix are another way that technology can help us to get active. My husband and I rarely see movies in the theatre anymore. We find that the seats are uncomfortable when you're sitting for so long. And getting up to stretch is generally frowned upon by the other movie-goers. Instead, we watch movies at home and press the pause button when we need a movement break.

Want to Hear About My First Movement Challenge?

Creating a movement challenge is a simple way to incorporate more non-exercise activity into your daily life. In early 2018, I created a five-day movement challenge called "Get off your butt!" I invited people to participate if they felt that their job kept them sedentary for most of the day. The premise was simple. Five one-minute video challenges were delivered to participants every morning, and a check-in email was sent at day's end to hold them accountable for that day's challenge. Participants watched an introductory video on a Sunday afternoon, and then every morning for one week, they received the instructions for the day. I will fill you in on exactly how the challenge works later in this section. First, though, let's review the results.

At the end of the week, I asked participants to complete a survey on the challenge. The first few questions asked them to explain how being sedentary impacted them. Here are some of their responses.

"I find I get constant aches and pains. My neck and shoulders are always tense, resulting in a lot of headaches."

"I feel like I'm losing part of my identity because I spent my 20s and 30s always on the go, playing sports."

"It makes me stiff and sore and contributes to generalized pain and achiness."

"It negatively affects my health and my mood."

Do any of these comments resonate with you? I hear these types of comments from people all the time.

When asked, "What worked well for you during this movement challenge?" responses were varied yet positive.

"My favourite part was putting my phone on the other side of the room. It resulted in less distraction (I didn't see that screen light up!), and it forced me to jump out of my seat every time the alarm rang."

"Reminders and having my colleagues interested and on board. More people and more accountability equals more fun!"

"The videos were only one minute long. That made it easy to watch them and get the info."

"Being accountable was good for me and [I liked] that there were different activities."

Participants loved the simple design of the movement challenges: short videos with easy-to-execute tasks. I deliberately created tasks that did not require complex skills or a high level of fitness.

As I mentioned earlier in the book, some participants in my test group incorrectly assumed they needed to "crush it" with these challenges. They wanted tougher options for the challenges; but that's not the point. These movement challenges are designed to break up sedentary behaviour patterns by encouraging you to get up and move when you've been sitting too long at work. Remember, a little movement goes a long way. And you're winning against yourself—your previously sedentary self. The goal is to get you up and moving, every day.

What Was Involved?

Let's review how the five-day movement challenge was structured. In the Sunday afternoon introductory video and email, participants received the following instructions, "For these challenges, you'll need a sticky note to record your daily progress. You can stick it to the side of your computer monitor or somewhere else in your line of sight when seated, so that it'll remind you to get up and complete the challenge. You'll be receiving some reminder emails throughout the day—I want you to try to complete the challenge multiple times that day. Once is great, but more is better.[72] At the end of the day, I'll ask you to snap a photo of your sticky note that you used to log your challenges, then email it to me. Hang on to all five sticky notes because at the end of the week, I'll ask you to take a photo of all of them together and send it to me."

Each daily challenge had a name that was linked to the movement it required and added a playful element to the activity:

> **Day 1** (Monday)—Reach for the sky
>
> **Day 2** (Tuesday)—Round and round the mulberry bush
>
> **Day 3** (Wednesday)—Time's running out
>
> **Day 4** (Thursday)—Shake it off

Day 5 (Friday)—I want YOU

The challenges were straightforward activities that anyone could complete:

- **Reach for the sky**: Stand up, reach both arms up to the ceiling, reach down toward the floor, and back to the middle. Repeat five times.

- **Round and round the mulberry bush**: Stand up and walk around your chair five times. Turn around and walk around it another five times. If your office or desk or cubicle space is too small for you to safely walk around your chair, look around and find a bigger space to use. Walk around your office; walk around the perimeter of the floor. Walk in both directions, to help your brain get unstuck from always walking in the same direction. Repeat six times throughout the day.

- **Time's running out**: Take out your smartphone, go to the clock or timer app. Set a timer for 30 minutes. Get up, walk across your office space, and put your phone up on a high shelf. Then go back to work. When the timer goes, you'll have to get up, walk over to it, and reach up to turn it off. And just like that, you added some great complex movement to your workday! Repeat this challenge seven times.

- **Shake it off**: Set your timer for 30 seconds, stand up, and "shake it off." When my kids were little, we used to call it "shaking your sillies out." Whatever works for you—just move in a relaxed way that gets lots of joints moving. Repeat this challenge eight times.
- **I want YOU**: Take your phone and snap a selfie of you pointing at the camera. Or take a photo of someone else pointing at the camera—someone who can help nudge you to move more. Or find a photo online of a hand pointing or a person pointing at you. Then go into your settings and make this image your lock screen on your phone. Every time you turn on your phone, you should see this image that is encouraging you to get up and move. And then, get up and move! Repeat this challenge 10 times.

Each day, the challenges grew more challenging, if you will. Not in complexity, but in the number of times participants were asked to complete the daily challenge:

> **Day 1** (Monday)—Reach for the sky: Repeat the challenge five times throughout the day.
>
> **Day 2** (Tuesday)—Round and round the mulberry bush: Repeat the challenge six times throughout the day.

Day 3 (Wednesday)—Time's running out:
Repeat the challenge seven times
throughout the day.

Day 4 (Thursday)—Shake it off: Repeat the
challenge eight times throughout the day.

Day 5 (Friday)—I want YOU: Repeat the
challenge 10 times throughout the day.

You may have noticed that the Day 5 challenge
jumped by two from the Day 4 challenge. Since the
Friday challenge was less complex than the others—
just get up and move—I believed participants could
add more iterations of the daily challenge. And since
most office workers are at home over the weekend, I
wanted them to have practiced more challenges
before taking a two-day break from their new routine
of adding simple movements to their workday.

In fact, though, many individuals who are mostly
sedentary at work, are also mostly sedentary at home.
One participant even acknowledged this fact as her
"aha" moment during the challenge:

"I realized that not only am I sitting a lot at work,
but I'm also doing it a lot in the evening. I come home
from work feeling exhausted, and then I tend to veg
on the couch reading as well, which just makes my
aches and pains worse!"

My mission with The Move More Institute™ is to
help people feel better by teaching them how to add

more movement—exercise and non-exercise activity—to their daily lives. And their lives don't end when they leave the office. Although I created this movement challenge with office workers in mind, I have had several retirees tell me that they too need help and nudges to be active and keep moving. It's not surprising, as older adults are the fastest-growing demographic on social media platforms like Facebook.[73] And more than half of the users are accessing social media with mobile devices.[74] Older adults hunched over their smartphones whilst they update their social media status—sounds like they have a lot more in common with their teenage grandchildren than the youngsters would like to admit![75]

Want to Create Your Own Movement Challenge?

Would you like to create your very own movement challenge? That's great news! You can take the details of the challenge I just shared with you and apply it to your life, or you can come up with other novel ways to add more movement. Here are a couple of ideas to switch it up.

Pick a washroom that's further away from your desk. If there's only one washroom, take a longer route to get there. You could call this challenge, "Take the long way home."

Do five chair squats every hour. You could call this challenge, "Get up, stand up." When you think about squats, I want you to think about the different ways you sit down, based on the seat you are using. If it's a comfy recliner, most people let gravity do the work and they don't engage their muscles as they let their bodies fall into the chair. But if you were to "drop" onto a toilet seat that way, you might slip off and hurt yourself. Instead, you lower your body with control. I want you to use that same level of control when you are doing your chair squats. And if your chair has wheels, please make sure the chair is wedged against a wall or furniture, or that you use a chair that won't move.

The sticky notes and emails serve as nudges to move, so make sure to include them in your challenge. You can also ask your colleagues if they would like to participate. Some participants in my challenge expressed interest in comparing their results to others, as a way to stay accountable. If you're competitive, the nudge of seeing other people's results might be just the ticket.

Even though one participant expressed interest in having a private Facebook group to compare results during the movement challenge, I purposely chose to keep social media out of the challenge. Too many people stay sedentary because they're spending so much time on social media. I wanted participants to stay focused on the challenge of moving more, not logging on to apps to read what others are doing.

You can use a free app like MailChimp to schedule emails to yourself and your co-competitors during the challenge. Alternatively, ask someone to check in with you throughout the day, or set reminders on your phone. There are lots of ways to nudge yourself toward moving more during a movement challenge; pick the one that works for you.

You know the drill: Time for a break! You've been sitting long enough; time to get up and move. Don't worry, I'm not going anywhere. I'll be right here, waiting for you. Now go move your beautiful body!

PART THREE:
THE ACTION PLAN

ADDING MOVEMENT
TO YOUR DAY

Solvitur Ambulando
(It is solved by walking).
— *Diogenes the Cynic (412-323 BCE)*

Are You a Helpful Harper, Sedentary Sam, or Fidget Finn?

I hope by now you understand the importance of adding small, sporadic bouts of movement to your daily life. My goal with this book and with The Move More Institute™ is to help you be more movement-oriented throughout the day, whether or not you also exercise in a more formal setting. The bottom line is that exercise and non-exercise activity are both important. But if you're doing neither, I would prefer you start by adding non-exercise activity to your life. You know, what I've called pre-exercise.

93

A great way to get moving is to become a Helpful Harper. As a child, I loved jumping up and fetching whatever the grown-ups in the room wanted. They were appreciative of my enthusiasm and I was glad to get away from the boring grown-up conversation. As a shy and introverted adult, I often offer to help at meetings, networking events, or in social settings as a way to avoid awkward small talk (awkward on my part, because my brain panics and forces my mouth to blurt out bizarre information).

Here are some ways you can be a Helpful Harper: An extra copy is needed for the latecomers to the meeting? I'll run to the photocopier and get it. Extra napkins are required and they're in the kitchen? Allow me. Someone needs to stand up and record comments on the flip chart? I'll do it. You get the idea—less sitting and more moving in a non-disruptive manner.

Whether you are at home full-time or you split your time between work, home, and supervising the activities of offspring or aging parents, you can add movement to your day in novel and inexpensive or free ways. I want you to evolve from being a Sedentary Sam to being a Fidget Finn; go from being a prolonger to a breaker. Let's recap these terms I introduced to you earlier.

A prolonger is someone who accumulates sedentary time in extended continuous bouts. A breaker is someone who accumulates sedentary time with frequent interruptions and in short bouts. Here's how I describe the differences to my clients: A prolonger is a Sedentary Sam, whilst a breaker is a Fidget Finn. Most people immediately recognize that being a Sedentary Sam is not a desirable end-state.

In the next sections, you'll see examples specific to home, work, and life outside of home and work that will demonstrate how you can be a Helpful Harper or a Fidget Finn. The goal is to evolve away from being a Sedentary Sam. I hope these samplings of everyday movement will inspire you to add more movement to your day.

Has Outsourcing Run Amok?

In the late 1990s, I was working in high tech. The flavour of the month was outsourcing. That meant hiring external experts to help you complete your project. You know the concept, you don't need to be an expert at everything, outsource some tasks to increase efficiency. So, outsourcing was always on the tip of everyone's tongue.

This included one colleague who talked about her activities on the home front: "I've outsourced my housecleaning," she told me.

Really? This same colleague regularly complained of having numerous aches and pains, difficulty sleeping, and general malaise. At the time, I thought about our cleaning regimen at home. Even then, my husband shared in the "homework" of maintaining a home. Although neither of us loved the actual work involved in housecleaning, we agreed that we preferred to save our money and get a little exercise in the process.

Don't get me wrong, it's not as if I loved cleaning the house. But it had to be done. And it was a classic example of killing two birds with one stone:

1. House needed to be cleaned; and
2. We needed to stay active at home and not become couch potatoes.

But there are ways to make it more fun. Yes, that's right, I said fun in relation to housework. Have you heard the saying, "Many hands make light work"? Teaming up to tackle the various jobs works wonders for getting the tasks accomplished, as does music.

During grad school, my sister and I shared an apartment. She was much neater than me, and she was constantly frustrated with my lack of interest in cleaning our apartment. She didn't love cleaning either, but she felt it needed to be done every week. So she started making mixed tapes[76] for housecleaning. The tapes had high-energy, motivating songs that would put us in a great mood while we washed the floors, dusted the living room, and cleaned the bathroom.

And it worked! She'd turn on the music, crank up the volume, and I'd emerge from my bedroom to do my share of the housework. Sometimes, we'd clean so vigorously to the music, we would both be short of breath and sweating.

Music makes any activity more enjoyable, especially tasks you don't really want to complete.

Can You Sneak in Some Movement?

A watched pot never boils, so step away from the stove and move! While you are waiting for that pot to boil, try adding some of these fun movements to your food prep time. Remember, I am not advocating that you add the activity while working in the kitchen. Please don't balance whilst using a knife or stirring a hot pot on the stove! I want you to do these things while you are standing around, waiting for the water to boil.

- **Pace**: Walk around the kitchen, and throw in a couple of loops around the kitchen table while you're at it;
- **Balance**: Work on your balance by standing on one leg for a minimum of 20 seconds. Hint: The timer is already set, so you can track your progress.
- **Alphabet**: Draw the letters of the alphabet with your foot. Try to draw as many letters as possible before you switch to the other foot. Hint: The letter M marks the halfway point of the 26 letters.

Are you caring for aging parents who could use a little more movement in their day? Want to help them get a spring back in their step? Maybe you need to help them out by sneaking in a little movement. The following story was shared with me when I was delivering a presentation about the importance of daily physical activity for older adults:

"My father likes to sit in his easy chair and eat cookies all afternoon. He places his cookie jar next to him on the side table. When we suggested that he get up and move around, he just waved us away with a laugh and then he reached for another cookie. So, we took his cookie jar and hid it. We placed it up on a high shelf in the other room. When he wants a cookie, he has to stand up, walk to the other room, and reach up to the highest shelf to get a cookie. Then, he walks around to eat it, so he doesn't leave any crumbs in his chair. He thinks we don't know that he knows where the cookie jar is, so he leaves it there and sneaks his daily cookie. Not only is he getting up and moving more, he's also eating fewer cookies."

Now that's what I call stealth activity!

Can You Be MORE Inefficient?

I used to be super-efficient, carrying a dizzying array of household items up or down the stairs—dirty dishes, clean kitchen towels, recycling, and more. Until the day I fell on the stairs. My arms were so full, that I couldn't see my feet and I actually missed the bottom step. Ouch.

In this case, being efficient with household chores was my downfall (pun intended). I decided that perhaps I should carry fewer things on the stairs and complete more trips instead. Extra trips definitely help increase your movement factor. And it's another way you can get exercise at home without needing special equipment. Stair climbers can cost upward of $3,000. Last time I checked, the stairs in my house were free to use. What about in your home? If you live in an apartment or condo, you've got even more stairs for the same low cost!

In my work as a mobile personal trainer, I sometimes see a client who lives on the 20th floor. The elevator in her building is V-E-R-Y slow. I timed it once and it took 10 minutes from when I pushed the button until it arrived in the lobby. So I started taking the stairs down after these house calls to get in a mini workout during my workday.

One day, I decided that maybe I should try to climb the stairs to her apartment, but halfway up I realized I would be completely out of breath for the training session. So I caught the elevator on the 10th floor, a compromise that still resulted in a mini-mini workout.

Do you putter in your home or garden? I believe puttering is a bit of a lost art, and it's a great way to get yourself moving. Even if you do outsource your housecleaning to someone else (a decision you already know I don't love, but that's your call) you still need to tidy up every day. You know, clear tables for meal prep and consumption, clean up the kitchen after a meal, put shoes and coats away. These are the little day-to-day tasks that can help you expend more energy without the need for a gym or structured workout.

For others, you may love to putter in your garden or tinker in your garage. You know, casual weeding

on a sunny day or reorganizing that tool drawer.
Every bit of movement helps, so putter away!

Do You Play with Your Pet?

Having pets can be a lot of fun. It can also be
physically demanding work that involves bending,
reaching, scooping, retrieving, playing, and walking.
Pet care is a great way to get you moving every day.
If you're not sure that you want the long-term
commitment of a pet, you can always look at fostering
animals or volunteering at a local shelter. Not too far
from our house, we regularly see volunteers walking
dogs that are training to become service dogs for
people with visual impairments.

One summer, we fostered three kittens for about
a month: three-month-old cuties from the same litter.
They all had an upper respiratory infection, or what's
known as a "kitty cold." When it was time for their
twice-daily medication, I had to catch them first.
They were not my biggest fans at that time. And since
they were incredibly active and mischievous, we
secured them in one room at night. My daughter and
I got quite the workout at bedtime because they saw
us coming and would flee. And having three kittens
meant twice-daily litter-box cleaning, which involves

a lot of stooping and scooping. I was moving a lot every day with the kittens in our home.

I hope you see that having pets helps you meet your daily physical activity needs. If you don't have your own pets, offer to pet sit for a friend or neighbour. That extra boost of activity will improve your day. And the non-humans will be thrilled to see you when you open the door to feed and play with them.

Have You Tried Our Obstacle Course?

Winters in Canada and many other parts of the northern hemisphere can be long and difficult. Frigid temperatures and even colder wind chill readings can sometimes make you a little stir crazy. When our children were younger and I was at home caring for them, some winters felt like they would never end. It was just too cold to play outside, in our opinion. But the kids and I would experience cabin fever.

One day, I came up with a solution: an indoor obstacle course. We moved furniture around to create a fun route throughout the house. We had to crawl under the table, walk around a series of stools and chairs, jump from one pillow-island to the next, walk upstairs, walk downstairs, and repeat. We had so much fun with the obstacle course that they even asked me to film them using it.[77]

One year, we were intrigued by blanket forts, so our courses were mostly army crawls. They were so much fun! And lots of movement and activity went into creating them and cleaning them up (although I was almost exclusively on my own when it came to the clean-up).

One particularly cold winter weekend, we didn't leave the house until school time Monday morning. By Sunday afternoon, my daughter and I were going a bit stir crazy, so we devised a simple "movement route": Walk around the dining room table five times, walk upstairs, walk the perimeter of our second level five times, walk downstairs, walk the other way around the table five times, and repeat 10 times. We had fun creating the movement challenge and completing it.

Have You Taken a SMOKE Break?

I've created a new mnemonic to get people moving more during the workday. I call it SMOKE: Sedentary & Movement Optional Kills Early. Think about it: Smokers move more than non-smokers at work. Isn't it ironic that while they're destroying their lungs, they're actually getting more physical activity than their non-smoking colleagues? It's still socially acceptable to go for a smoke break at work. And because of indoor no-smoking laws, they have to leave the building to do so. Somehow it is less socially acceptable to leave your desk to take a walk. But we know that incorporating more movement in our lives is not optional. A sedentary lifestyle leads to premature aging and death. We NEED to move more throughout the day.

So tell your boss you're taking a healthy SMOKE break for your body and your mind. And then get up from your desk and move. Go for a walk, stretch your arms up to the sky, twist and turn as you re-energize yourself head to toe. Not everything in our lives needs to be all or nothing. Just because you can't make it to the gym doesn't mean you can't move. And even if you do go to the gym, you should still incorporate those snacks of movement into your daily life.

Do You Have Space to Pace?

Stuck on hold? Don't just sit there! Get up and find some space to pace. It can make that time on hold feel much less frustrating. Let me give you an example.

One day, I had a banking issue and required assistance from my bank. I walked to my local branch, stood in line, explained my dilemma to the teller, and was told to call the 1-800 number. He pointed to a phone in the branch and said, "You can call from there. You know, in case they have questions for me." The phone was a retro-style landline, complete with a phone cord that connected the handset to the base. I dialled the number and waited; the automated voice told me the wait time was at least 20 minutes.

After three minutes of waiting on hold (in which many other banking customers approached me with questions because they thought I worked there), I gave up and walked home. If I was going to be on hold that long, I preferred using my speakerphone so I could move around.

Once at home, I dialled the 1-800 number again, switched my cordless phone to speaker mode, and got up from my desk. Whilst on hold, I cleaned the kitchen, put away some boots in the front hall, and began dusting the house. By the time my call was answered, I was in a much better frame of mind to speak with the person on the other end of the line. I don't know about you, but sitting and waiting on hold can increase my blood pressure and make me moody and testy—not the best way to speak with someone whose job it is to help resolve your issue.

You can do this in meetings as well. After attending one of my "Sit Less, Move More" workshops, someone told me: "Today, while I was in four hours of teleconference meetings, I got up and moved around. Thank you for the tips, [I'm] already making changes in my day!"

How Can Employers Help You Move More at Work?

If you're an employer and you're concerned about your employees' physical inactivity levels, this section is for you. You'll remember that, for nudges to ensure behaviour change, they need to be inexpensive and easy to implement.[78] You can start by having your IT department change employees' printer settings: Instead of the default printer being closest to their desk, make the default the printer that is farthest from them. Just like that, you get your staff up and walking more.

To encourage the use of stairs over elevators, I have several tips.

I often look for stairs first when I enter a building; however, they can sometimes be difficult to locate. And yet the elevator is typically in plain sight. Paint footsteps on the floor or along the wall that leads from the elevator to the stairwell. Our local children's hospital uses footprints of different animals to guide visitors to various departments. They appear along the wall from the main entrance to guide you, and they are adorable to look at!

Make the stairwells more visually appealing. Most stairwells are boring and grey. Recently, a friend in Boston shared with me a video of a painted stairwell. It was visually appealing and made me want to use their stairs. Artwork by graffiti artists works well in these large-scale spaces. When I worked in high tech in the 1990s, the Nortel office in Brampton, Ontario, had hired graffiti artists to paint the large walls leading to the loading docks. It became a favourite stop during tours of the facility.

Another way to make the stairs more appealing is to post trivia questions or fun facts on the walls. If you choose the trivia option, it can become an office challenge to see who answers the most questions correctly in a set amount of time.

Try painting a face, or even just eyes, on the door to the stairwell. People respond to the illusion of eye contact from these still images. Remember the Uncle Sam posters, "I want YOU," that were used in iconic American recruitment campaigns? The figure of Uncle Sam was pointing at whoever was looking at the poster. They work. The painting on the stairwell door could include a speech bubble with a statement like, "Will you take the stairs with me?"

If staff are reluctant to use the stairs (some people don't want to feel sweaty at work) you can post fun challenges for them at the elevator or in the elevator: Balance on one leg for 20 seconds, or see how many letters of the alphabet you can write with your foot or leg before the elevator arrives. This is about fun movement that anyone can do.

And don't discount the importance of social influence. Encourage leaders to get up and take stretch breaks during meetings; it will make it appear less risky for staff to do the same. If employees see senior management using the stairs instead of the elevator, they may be more likely to follow suit. A statement by the elevators like, "Most people like you in the office use the stairs," will go a long way to encouraging more movement at work.[79]

When IT staff are updating printer settings on employee computers, have them also change the desktop screensavers to be an image that encourages physical activity. Some ideas include footprints, stairs, or people walking. Even a scrolling sentence like, "Don't forget to get up and stretch; many of your colleagues are doing it," can help increase social influence to get staff moving more. Your IT department can also set pop-up reminders on employees' computers to prompt them to get up from their desks at regular intervals.

You know the drill: Time for a break! You've been sitting long enough; time to get up and move. Don't worry, I'm not going anywhere. I'll be right here, waiting for you. Now go move your beautiful body!

ADDING MOVEMENT WHEN YOU'RE OUT & ABOUT

I like to get outside every day, breath in the fresh air, and feel my muscles working. If my muscles feel tired at the end of the day, it was a good day.
— C.D., 83 years old

Do You Need a Nudge?

When you're going about your daily life, there are many ways you can add more movement. The key is to nudge yourself toward a moderate amount of inconvenience so that you're required to move more. And perhaps you'll think of other ways that non-exercise activity can sneak into your life!

Why Don't You Eschew the Drive-Through?

One of the ways our environment discourages physical activity is the drive-through window.

Whether it's a drive-through coffee shop, fast-food joint, pharmacy, or bank ATM, it's a convenience that equates to short-term gain, long-term pain in the form of deteriorating your physical health. (And I'm not actually convinced this so-called time-saver actually saves any time at all.) Why not be good to your body and park the car and walk into the business establishment in question? Seriously, you'll be better off with the added movement.

And remember, there's always a spot at the end of the lot. Everyone else wants to park as close to the door as possible. Well, not everyone. I prefer to park further away and walk more. As I'm walking through the parking lot, I see many frustrated drivers circling close to the door, looking for the closest spot. Save yourself some aggravation and just head to the far end of the parking lot. You'll get some additional physical activity with that extra-long walk and you'll be less stressed when you walk through the doors and begin to fight the crowds of shoppers.

Or you can take it a step further and leave your car at home. When you have to run errands, do you have to hop in your car and race from one destination to the next? Next time, take a few moments to plan, and walk your errands instead. Or at least, walk a few of them. The other day, I needed to pick up a book at the library AND get more milk. So, I walked a two-kilometre loop. And the second half of my walk included a suitcase carry with four litres of milk. That milk jug weighs just over nine pounds.

Functional fitness like the suitcase carry is a great exercise to strengthen your oblique abdominal muscles, improve your grip strength, and get muscles engaged from your forearm up to your shoulder and back. That walk with the heavy milk will help you the next time you have to sprint through an airport with luggage. I hope this explanation didn't make my suggestion too "fitness-y" for you. Functional fitness just refers to exercises that help you train your body to do everyday activities with ease and without pain. Functional fitness improves strength, trains your muscles to work together, improves your balance, and reduces the risk of a fall. But now I'll get back to talking about non-exercise movement.

When you finally get to the grocery store, a supercentre like Walmart or Target, or a large-scale hardware store like Home Depot, do you stand in line to have your purchases scanned and packed by a human, or do you use the self-scan checkout? I prefer to use the self-scan because it allows me to add more movement to my shopping experience. Think about it: You're lifting, reaching, twisting, and turning. It's a great mini workout, especially if you've got heavier items like a 10-pound bag of flour (my husband bakes a lot). It's another example of free exercise.

Do You Use the Heel-Toe Express?

I usually arrive at business meetings in my running shoes. I love the feature on most mapping apps that allows you to choose mode of transportation when you're mapping your route. I try to choose the heel-toe express—aka walking—as much as possible. If the estimated travel time is less than one hour, it's walking time for me! It's physical activity that doesn't cost anything and that's easy to fit into the day—a win-win in my opinion.

In my teens and twenties, I walked everywhere. Sure, I had a bus pass, and I used to wait at the bus stop. But the only thing I disliked more than waiting in line to purchase my monthly bus pass was standing and waiting for a bus. So I would check the posted bus schedule (this was in the dark ages before we had apps at our fingertips for everything) and then I would check my watch. I would also peer down the road, looking for the next bus. If I couldn't see the bus, I would start to walk, figuring I could make it to the next stop before the bus arrived.

I would repeat this cycle at the next stop. Eventually, I would be within two or three stops of my destination and I was still walking. The only logical decision at this point was to keep walking because I didn't want to be one of those people who only rides the bus for two stops. It was typically around the time I decided to walk the entire way that the bus would finally drive by. And more often than not, I was between bus stops anyway.

After grad school, it was time for me to enter the workforce like a grown-up. I had two key criteria that had to be met in my job search: distance and facilities. Let me explain why.

One of my jobs during grad school was a one-hour bus ride each way. I decided to switch to cycling but it didn't save me any time. It was still one hour each way, and the roads were dangerous for cyclists. I was relieved when my work term was finished and I vowed to find a job closer to home, or at least along a bike path! My first criteria was being able to get to the office in a reasonable amount of time by cycling, jogging, or walking.

Having decided to choose active transportation as much as possible, my second criteria was having showers on-site. Nobody would want to sit beside me in a meeting if I smelled of sweat every day. Even walking to work could induce sweating during the dog days of summer.

When I finally did get a car (which was gifted to me by my great aunt) I preferred to leave it at home. Most of my employers charged a fee for a parking pass and the cost of filling the tank wasn't cheap either. As a research assistant working on funded health-promotion research projects, I wasn't exactly raking in the dough, so I didn't appreciate having to spend money on a car I didn't even like driving. As a result, I stuck with my two-wheel, two-feet philosophy of commuting.

Are You a Fair-Weather Walker?

During the 1990s tech boom, I worked as a human resources consultant in high tech. As a thank-you for the long hours we spent completing one project, a colleague and I were sent on a spa weekend together. We shared the accommodations, and the late fall evenings involved wine and conversation in front of a roaring fire. She told me stories about her hiking adventures, but since my husband and I were urban adventurers, I had no stories to share—none that interested her, that is.

At one point, she lamented that the start of winter meant her hiking would be curtailed. She said, "I wish there was a way I could keep hiking all winter long."

"There is," I replied. "It's called mall walking."

She nearly fell off the couch as she spat out a mouthful of wine, laughing at my suggestion. But I wasn't kidding. At the time, mall walking for seniors wasn't a big thing, at least not where I lived. Now, it is very popular with seniors' groups. And it's another free way to exercise. It's a weatherproof walk that can be done at any time of year, wind chill or humidex be damned.

Another great way to enjoy a weatherproof walk is to visit your local museum. When our first born was 18 months old, we purchased a family membership to our local museums.[80] The membership came as a bundle, so we could visit three museums: the Canada Agriculture and Food Museum, the Canada Aviation and Space Museum, and the Canada Science and Technology Museum. We had a small house with no basement and a rambunctious toddler who couldn't manoeuvre the icy sidewalks that winter. So, I took him to a museum and let him walk or run from one exhibit to the next. It helped keep us both sane during our long winters. Although the museums are not a free form of exercise, they are indeed weatherproof walks. And I still love visiting them for an educational and inspiring walk.

You know the drill: Time for a break! You've been sitting long enough; time to get up and move. Don't worry, I'm not going anywhere. I'll be right here, waiting for you. Now go move your beautiful body!

WHAT'S STOPPING YOU FROM MOVING MORE?

If I'd known I was going to live this long, I'd
have taken better care of myself.
— Eubie Blake

At this point, I'm hoping you're excited about the
ways you can add more movement to your day. I
have given you many examples on how to get active,
but I am also realistic about your potential barriers[81] —
excuses and external interferences that can impact
your ability to adopt new behaviours.

Below are some examples of potential internal
and external barriers.[82] Internal barriers refer to you
and your excuses for not being more physically
active. Remember, this is not about judging you; we
are simply identifying potential roadblocks. External
barriers refer to the world outside your brain and

body, and how it might impact your ability to be more physically active.

Here are some examples of barriers to being physically active.

You
Lack of time
Lack of energy or motivation
No knowledge of exercises
Dislike of sweating
Weight

Social
Commitments with family or friends
Work obligations

Environmental
Lack of access
Safety concerns
Bad weather
Cost
No shower

Do you see a pattern at all with these lists? If not, let me help you: These potential barriers should not impact your goal of adding non-exercise activity to your day. Let's go through the list together based on everything you've learned in this book. You can use these suggestions to overcome barriers or come up with your own. There are no right or wrong answers. The goal of this chapter is to anticipate roadblocks and pre-emptively remove them.

1. You

Lack of time: If you don't have time to move more, do you have time to be sick or injured? The snacks of movement I've described in this book can easily be squeezed into your busy day. I'm not talking about a time-laden location change where you pack your gym bag, drive to a facility, change your clothes, exercise, remove your workout clothes, shower, change again, and drive back to work or home. I'm referring to sporadic bouts of movement that will fit into your schedule and enhance your day. No matter who you are, you can take 15 seconds to stand up, reach for the sky and sit back down again.

Lack of energy or motivation: If you move more, you will feel better. Based on my experience as a personal trainer, I know that this improved sense of well-being will re-energize you and motivate you to start and keep moving more. And until that happens, you can incorporate tangible pats on the back to keep you motivated, just as Janet, a long-time regular at my group fitness classes, does. Janet uses stars on her calendar: "This is my star system. One gold star for attending class and another for walking there and back. I find it rewarding to look back over the month and see all the stars. Whatever motivates a person! Right?" That's right, Janet! So, grab a pack of stars or stickers and start rewarding your new behaviour.

If the stickers don't cut it, try this: I am so proud of you for sticking with your new behaviour. You're doing a great job and I'm doing a happy dance to celebrate your success. Dance with me!

No knowledge of exercises: Stand up. Walk around. Bend down to pet your dog. Reach up to put away that cup. Do any of these instructions sound to you like fancy exercises? Nope. They are just natural, everyday movement that your body needs and craves. There are no specialized exercises or workouts to remember, just movement—any movement. Please.

Dislike of sweating: There is no sweating involved with the non-exercise activity I'm prescribing. No change of clothes required, no sweating, and no shower needed.

Weight: Of some types of exercise, individuals may say, "I'm too heavy, I can't do that." But you are already doing the types of movement and activity that I am suggesting because you are moving about the world in your daily life. I just want you to get out of your chair and do them more.

2. Social

Commitments with family or friends: There's always a way to include others in your movement objectives. If you have to drive your child to their after-school activity, make a commitment to walk around while they're at their session. If you need to meet your brother or sister to talk about family business, suggest to them that you add a walk to the talk. If they would prefer to stay indoors, pace around the table whilst talking, or be a Helpful Harper and get up whenever someone needs something. If you are caring for your grandchildren, get on the floor and play with them. If your friends want to meet up for drinks, walk to the restaurant; if you're meeting at someone's home, suggest a fun playlist and begin with a dance-off. There are many ways that your newfound commitment to move more can be incorporated into social commitments. Being active with others will make you feel even better, especially since the movement can be adapted for all fitness levels.

Work obligations: Much of the non-exercise activity I am prescribing should happen during your workday. Remember SMOKE breaks? That means Sedentary & Movement Optional Kills Early. Tell your boss you're taking a moment for a healthy SMOKE break. I suspect they will encourage you to do it more often, and they just may join you. In a survey by Towers Watson, employers identified physical inactivity as the second most important lifestyle risk factor affecting their workforce.[83]

3. Environmental

Lack of access: No gym close to your home or work? No access is needed. I'm not suggesting you join a gym. I'm suggesting you get off your butt and move around!

Safety concerns or bad weather: I have lumped safety and weather together because they relate to exercising outside, possibly at night if your schedule is very full during the day, or if you live or work in a sketchy neighbourhood. While there are many benefits to getting outside for a walk, including fresh air and a boost of Vitamin D if it is sunny, the bulk of the natural movement I am suggesting in this book takes place indoors. Remember, too much sitting for long periods is the problem we are trying to solve. I want to nudge you to get up and move around more often, not nudge you to go out and run a marathon. You're not going outside during an ice storm. You're not donning your runners to hit the pavement in the dark. You are adding these bouts of movement during your daily activities. So, no scene change is required.

Cost: You don't need special clothing, fancy equipment, or an expensive gym membership to add non-exercise activity to your day. It's free, so cost is never a problem with natural movement.

No shower: Again, no sweating involved, so no shower is needed. Just get up and move more.

Let's recap: No special equipment, change of clothing, fancy exercise sequences, or location changes are required to just get off your butt and move more. If you aren't already there, I hope you have an "aha" moment as this last statement sinks in.

And I have one more thing to say: Just. One. Thing. You have the power to feel better. Start with just one thing you can do differently right now. Just one thing, that's all I'm asking. I have given you many ideas in this book, please take just one thing you have learned and apply it right now.

If you move more, you will feel better. Guaranteed.

You know the drill: Time for a break! You've been sitting long enough; time to get up and move. Don't worry, I'm not going anywhere. I'll be right here, waiting for you. Now go move your beautiful body!

APPENDIX: MORE FROM THE MOVE MORE INSTITUTE™

MOVEMENT COACHING

What is movement coaching all about? It is unlike anything you've ever experienced. It's movement training that teaches you to embrace the natural movement patterns your body craves, delivered in an online course that will help you change your behaviour from "mostly sedentary" to "active mover." Currently, I offer five online courses through The Move More Institute™. You can read about them in the following pages or visit my website for more information: www.themovemoreinstitute.com. All of these courses can be self-guided: you get the videos, newsletters, homework, and other material, and work at your own pace. Some of them also have a coach-guided option where we have regular check-ins via video chat or text message. And once you've registered and paid for the course, you have lifetime access to the videos.

3 DAYS TO BETTER BALANCE

You don't have to be elderly to be concerned about your balance. We all need good balance to safely move around our world on a daily basis. But have you ever thought about it? Among adults, poor balance can lead to injury. The course 3 Days to Better Balance will help you improve body awareness, strengthen your brain-body connection, and learn how to take off your shoes and get those feet activated!

Each day, you'll receive a video and an email from me; both will be chock full of tips and exercises that will help you improve your balance. You'll also get an opportunity to chat with me via text. I'll answer your questions and keep you accountable for the goal of better balance.

Topics

Day 1: Your balance system: visual, vestibular & proprioception

Day 2: Active standing

Day 3: The mechanics of walking

Bonus! Walking backwards for posture and balance

BALANCE 2.0: PROGRESSIONS IN MOTION

Remember worrying about your balance as a child? You didn't, did you? You moved about your world in a carefree manner. This course will help you reclaim your balance and bring you back to that way of living. Balance 2.0 will help you improve control of your body whilst moving, increase your coordination, and prevent injury.

Each day, you'll receive a video that is full of tips and exercises to help you improve your balance. You'll also get an opportunity to chat with me via text. I'll answer your questions and keep you accountable for the goal of better balance.

Topics

Day 1: Balance progressions

Day 2: The power of lateral movement

Day 3: Complex moves & core strength

GET OFF YOUR BUTT! 5-DAY MOVEMENT CHALLENGE

You've read about my movement challenge in the book, but perhaps you want the accountability of regular check-ins from me. This course will get you to move more during your workday.

Daily challenges are delivered by video, but don't worry because they're short and sweet at one minute each. You'll get regular nudges throughout the day to keep you on track, plus an end-of-day check-in to record your progress.

Topics

Day 1: Reach for the sky

Day 2: Round and round the mulberry bush

Day 3: Time's running out

Day 4: Shake it off

Day 5: I want YOU

ADD MOVEMENT AT WORK

This six-week online course will teach you how to add small bouts of non-exercise activity to your workday. The course includes weekly newsletters and videos that will give you quick and easy exercises to do at your desk, as well as tips to add more movement during the day. The videos will lead you through the exercises (the what), and the newsletters will delve into the importance of the movement (the why).

Weekly Topics

Week 1: Active sitting—engage more muscles when sitting

Week 2: Active standing—engage more
 muscles when standing
Week 3: Fingers and toes, hands and feet
Week 4: Stretch your neck, shoulders and
 back
Week 5: Getting up from your desk, office
 squats
Week 6: Fidget!

You can choose a self-guided or coach-guided program. If you choose the self-guided program, you'll work through the exercises on your own. If you select the coach-guided program, you'll also have a weekly video chat with me. We'll review the exercises and see how you're doing with incorporating them into your workday.

MOVE MORE! COACHING FOR BEHAVIOUR CHANGE

I can help you create new habits to add more movement to your daily life. That's what movement coaching is all about.

You CAN teach an old dog new tricks! Have you been told that you should sit less and move more? It's a common theme with many health and fitness professionals. If you're only relying on willpower to change your behaviour, you may fall short of your goal.

With my unique combination of skills and experience—two social psychology degrees, a background in health promotion research, and almost 10 years in the fitness industry—I have created a groundbreaking course that will be delivered right to your inbox.

Weekly Topics

Week 1: Do you believe you can change?

Week 2: Creating external rewards

Week 3: Your behaviour—activity clocks and the three Ds

Week 4: Prolonger or breaker

Week 5: The habit loop

Week 6: Experiment with rewards

Week 7: Cue awareness training

Week 8: Create a plan

Week 9: What are your disruptors?

Week 10: Your inconvenience set-up rating

Week 11: I'm too busy

Week 12: Adopting the new behaviour

You can choose from a self-guided or coach-guided program. Each week, you'll receive a newsletter, a video, and a homework assignment. If you choose the self-guided program, you'll work through the exercises on your own. If you select the coach-guided program, you'll also have a weekly video chat with me. We'll review your homework assignment and discuss your progress.

You know the drill: Time for a break! You've been sitting long enough; time to get up and move. Don't worry, I'm not going anywhere. I'll be right here, waiting for you. Now go move your beautiful body!

ENDNOTES

[1] Meik Wiking, *The Little Book of Lykke: The Danish Search for the World's Happiest People* (Canada: Penguin Random House, 2017): 144–145.

[2] World Health Organization, *Global Health Risks: Mortality and Burden of Disease Attributable to Selected Major Risk* (Geneva: World Health Organization, 2009), http://www.who.int/healthinfo/global_burden_disease/GlobalHealthRisks_report_full.pdf.

[3] *Cholesterol: The Great Bluff*, TV Ontario (documentary created and posted on the TVO website), accessed July 10, 2017, http://tvo.org/video/documentaries/cholesterol-the-great-bluff.

[4] World Health Organization, *Fact Sheet on Physical Activity*, http://www.who.int/topics/physical_activity/en/.

[5] Yasuhiko Kubota et al., "TV viewing and incident venous thromboembolism: The Atherosclerotic Risk in Communities Study," *Journal of Thrombosis and Thrombolysis*, 45, no. 3, (April

2018): 353–359, https://doi.org/10.1007/s11239-018-1620-7.

[6] Mark S. Tremblay et al., "Sedentary Behaviour Research Network (SBRN) – Terminology Consensus Project process and outcome," *International Journal of Behavioural Nutrition and Physical Activity* 14 (June 10, 2017): 75, https://doi.org/10.1186/s12966-017-0525-8. Reprinted with permission.

[7] A description of the network from their website: "The Sedentary Behaviour Research Network (SBRN) is the only organization for researchers and health professionals which focuses specifically on the health impact of sedentary behaviour." http://www.sedentarybehaviour.org/about/. Reprinted with permission.

[8] Amy Cuddy, *Presence: Bringing Your Boldest Self to Your Biggest Challenges* (New York: Little, Brown and Company: 2015), 226–228.

[9] David W Dunstan et al., "Too Much Sitting and Metabolic Risk—Has Modern Technology Caught Up with Us?" *European Endocrinology*, 6 (2010):19–23, http://doi.org/10.17925/EE.2010.06.00.19.

[10] Bonnie Berkowitz, "The Health Hazards of Sitting," *The Washington Post*, January 20, 2014, http://apps.washingtonpost.com/g/page/national/the-health-hazards-of-sitting/750/.

[11] Berkowitz, *The Health Hazards of Sitting*.

[12] Robert Wood, "Why Seniors Fall," *Electronics Caregiver* (March

29, 2012), https://www.youtube.com/watch?v=T5x6kTrwgYw. Reprinted with permission.

[13] Miranda Esmonde-White, *Aging Backwards: 10 Years Younger, 10 Years Lighter, 30 Minutes A Day* (Toronto: Random House Canada, 2014), 37.

[14] George Cranston, "Muscle Atrophy: Symptoms, Causes and Treatments," Health Guidance (blog), January 24, 2012, http://www.healthguidance.org/entry/14727/1/muscle-atrophy-symptoms-causes-and-treatments.html.

[15] James A. Levine, "Nonexercise activity thermogenesis (NEAT): environment and biology," *American Journal of Physiology, Endocrinology & Metabolism*, 288, no. 1 (January 2005): E285, https://www.ncbi.nlm.nih.gov/pubmed/15102614.

[16] Katy Bowman, *Move Your DNA: Restore Your Health Through Natural Movement* (United States of America: Propriometrics Press, 2014), 21. Reprinted with permission.

[17] Daniel Wolpert, "The real reason for brains," *TED Talk* (July 2011), http://www.ted.com/talks/daniel_wolpert_the_real_reason_for_brains.

[18] Jack P. Callaghan et al., "Is Standing the Solution to Sedentary Office Work?" *Ergonomics in Design* 23, no. 3 (July 21, 2015): 20-24, https://doi.org/10.1177/1064804615585412.

[19] Ian Janssen. "Health Care Costs of Physical Inactivity in Canadian Adults." *Applied Physiology, Nutrition, and Metabolism* 37, no. 4 (2012): 803–806.

[20] World Health Organization, *Fact Sheet on Physical Activity*,

http://www.who.int/topics/physical_activity/en/. Reprinted with permission.

[21] Hayley Wickenheiser, "We must move more to improve Canadians' health," *Ottawa Citizen*, March 15, 2017, http://ottawacitizen.com/opinion/columnists/wickenheiser-we-must-move-more-to-improve-canadians-health.

[22] Fares Bounajm, Thy Dinh, and Louis Thériault, *Moving Ahead: The Economic Impact of Reducing Physical Inactivity and Sedentary Behaviour* (Ottawa: The Conference Board of Canada, 2014): 15, http://sportmatters.ca/sites/default/files/content/moving_ahead_economic_impact_en.pdf.

[23] Canadian Society for Exercise Physiology, *Canadian Physical Activity Guidelines for Adults—18–64 years*, (first viewed October 10, 2017), http://www.csep.ca/CMFiles/Guidelines/CSEP_PAGuidelines_adults_en.pdf.

[24] CSEP, *Canadian Physical Activity Guidelines*.

[25] Rachel C. Colley et al., "Physical activity of Canadian adults: Accelerometer results from the 2007 to 2009 Canadian Health Measures Survey," *Health Reports* 22, no. 1 (January 2011): 4, http://www.statcan.gc.ca/pub/82-003-x/2011001/article/11396-eng.pdf.

[26] Colley, "Physical activity of Canadian adults", 4.

[27] Carol Ewing Garber et al., "Quantity and Quality of Exercise for Developing and Maintaining Cardiorespiratory, Musculoskeletal, and Neuromotor Fitness in Apparently

Healthy Adults: Guidance for Prescribing Exercise," *Medicine & Science in Sports & Exercise* 43, no. 7 (July 2011): 1334–1359, https://journals.lww.com/acsm-msse/Fulltext/2011/07000/Quantity_and_Quality_of_Exercise_for_Developing.26.aspx.

[28] Nabil Ebraheim, "Causes and Treatments of Low Back Pain," *The Huffington Post Blog* (October 7, 2016), https://www.huffingtonpost.com/nabil-ebraheim-md/causes-and-treamnet-of-lo_b_12386470.html.

[29] Stephanie Watson, "10 Ways to Manage Low Back Pain at Home," *WebMD* (March 12, 2014), https://www.webmd.com/back-pain/features/manage-low-back-pain-home#1.

[30] Watson, "Manage Low Back Pain."

[31] Nadine E. Foster et al., "Prevention and treatment of low back pain: evidence, challenges, and promising directions," *The Lancet* (March 2018), https://doi.org/10.1016/S0140-6736(18)30489-6.

[32] Thanks to Brad Lafortune, Owner & Physiotherapist at Function Physiotherapy, for permission to share elements our conversation from March 1, 2018. You can find out more about Brad and his clinic here: www.fxnphysio.com.

[33] Pedro F. Saint-Maurice et al., "Moderate-to-Vigorous Physical Activity and All-Cause Mortality: Do Bouts Matter?" *Journal of the American Heart Association* (March 22, 2018), https://doi.org/10.1161/JAHA.117.007678.

[34] "'I'm older than the Academy': Eva Marie Saint hands out Oscar at age 93," CTV News, March 4, 2018,

https://www.ctvnews.ca/i-m-older-than-the-academy-eva-marie-saint-hands-out-oscar-at-age-93-1.3828591.

[35] Ryan Halvorson, "Exercise Doesn't Have To Be Strenuous To Be Effective," IDEA Health & Fitness Association (blog), April 31, 2018, http://www.ideafit.com/fitness-library/exercise-doesnrsquot-have-to-be-strenuous-to-be-effective.

[36] Eric Jensen, "Teaching with the brain in mind," chap. 4 in *Movement and learning*, 2nd ed. (Alexandria: Association for Supervision and Curriculum Development, 2005), http://www.ascd.org/publications/books/104013/chapters/Movement-and-Learning.aspx.

37 You'll read more about these challenges in the chapter, "Creating a Movement Challenge."

[38] James A. Levine, "Nonexercise activity thermogenesis (NEAT): environment and biology," *American Journal of Physiology, Endocrinology & Metabolism*, 288, no. 1 (January 2005): E285, https://www.ncbi.nlm.nih.gov/pubmed/15102614.

[39] James A. Levine and Selene Yeager, *Move a Little, Lose A Lot. New NEAT Science Reveals How to Be Thinner, Happier, and Smarter* (New York: Crown Publishing, 2009).

[40] Christian von Loeffelholz, "The Role of Non-exercise Activity Thermogenesis in Human Obesity," Edited by LJ De Groot et al. *Endotext: Comprehensive Free Online Endocrinology Book* (South Dartmout: MDText, 2004, https://www.ncbi.nlm.nih.gov/books/NBK279077/.

[41] Joan Vernikos, Sitting Kills, *Moving Heals. How Simple Everyday*

Movement Will Prevent Pain, Illness, and Early Death—and Exercise Alone Won't (Fresno: Quill Driver Books, 2011), 36. Reprinted with permission.

[42] David W Dunstan et al., "Too Much Sitting and Metabolic Risk—Has Modern Technology Caught Up with Us?" *European Endocrinology* 6 (2010):19–23; http://doi.org/10.17925 /EE.2010.06.00.19

[43] Vernikos, *Sitting Kills*, 36.

[44] Rachel C. Colley, Isabelle Michaud and Didier Garriguet, "Reallocating time between sleep, sedentary and active behaviours: Associations with obesity and health in Canadian adults," *Health Reports* 29, no. 4 (April 18, 2018) http://www.statcan.gc.ca/pub/82-003-x/2018004/article/54951-eng.htm.

[45] "No! That is my food!"

[46] ParticipACTION (website), accessed October 3, 2016, https://www.participaction.com/en-ca.

[47] ParticipACTION (website), Canada 150 Play List, accessed October 22, 2016, https://www.participaction.com/en-ca/programs/participaction-150-play-list/about.

[48] For more information on Essentrics® and Classical Stretch™, visit http://essentrics.com.

[49] Miranda Esmonde-White, *Aging Backwards: 10 Years Younger, 10 Years Lighter, 30 Minutes A Day* (Toronto: Random House Canada, 2014).

[50] Miranda Esmonde-White, *Forever Painless: Lasting Relief Through Gentle Movement* (Toronto: Random House Canada, 2016).

[51] ParticipACTION (website), Fitness Activities, accessed April 3, 2018, https://www.participaction.com/en-ca/programs/participaction-150-play-list/activities/fitness-activities?q=var/www/html/www.participaction.com/fr-ca/programmes/le-palmarès-150-de-participaction/activities/mise-en-forme.

[52] "Rating of Perceived Exertion Scale," *Productive Fitness*, accessed October 10, 2016, http://www.productivefitness.com/ratingofPerceivedexertion.aspx. Reprinted with permission.

[53] Michelle E. Mlinac and Michelle C. Feng, "Assessment of Activities of Daily Living, Self-Care, and Independence," *Archives of Clinical Neuropsychology*, 31, no. 5 (September 1, 2016), https://doi.org/10.1093/arclin/acw049.

[54] Time of Care Online Medicine Notebook (website), DEATH SHAFT: ADL & IADL Mnemonics, accessed May 1, 2018, https://www.timeofcare.com/adl-mnemonic/.

[55] Excerpt from a telephone interview with Patrick Smith, conducted on April 20, 2018.

[56] Nicola Twilley, "A Pill To Make Exercise Obsolete: What If A Pill Could Give You All The Benefits Of Exercise?" *The New Yorker*, November 6, 2017, https://www.newyorker.com/magazine/2017/11/06/a-pill-to-make-exercise-obsolete.

[57] James A. Levine, "Nonexercise activity thermogenesis (NEAT): environment and biology," *American Journal of Physiology, Endocrinology & Metabolism,* 288, no. 1 (January 2005): E285, https://www.ncbi.nlm.nih.gov/pubmed/15102614.

[58] Marc T. Hamilton et al., "Too little exercise and too much sitting: Inactivity physiology and the need for new recommendations on sedentary behavior," *Current Cardiovascular Risk Reports* 2 (July 2008): 292, https://doi.org/10.1007/s12170-008-0054-8.

[59] There are many behaviour change models, too many to summarize in this book. The models I have adopted in my practice are more complex than what I describe here, but the principles are the same. If you're keen to read more, I have included additional references that you can consult for more information.

[60] No, the cat didn't manage to "retrain" me to feed her earlier. In fact, she now sleeps in later; I think she realizes that the food is more likely to be in her bowl if she waits a little longer.

[61] Charles Duhigg, *The Power of Habit—Why We Do What We Do in Life and Business* (New York: Random House, 2012).

[62] Visit http://charlesduhigg.com to download free resources on changing a habit.

[63] Coaching for behaviour change is a more involved process that is beyond the scope of this book. But you can always visit http://themovemoreinstitute.com if you would like to work with me on changing your behaviour.

[64] Tiny Habits website, accessed February 12, 2017, http://tinyhabits.com.

[65] *What About Bob?* Description from the Internet Movie Database's website, accessed January 3, 2017, https://www.imdb.com/title/tt0103241/.

[66] Richard H. Thaler and Cass R. Sunstein, *Nudge: Improving Decisions About Health, Wealth, and Happiness*, (New York: Penguin Books, 2008).

[67] Ian Herbert, "Exercising Judgement: The Psychology of Fitness," *Association for Psychological Science* (January 1, 2008), https://www.psychologicalscience.org/observer/exercising-judgement-the-psychology-of-fitness.

[68] "The surprising way to feel less busy," ParticipACTION (blog), June 9, 2017, https://www.participaction.com/en-ca/peptalk/lifestyle-culture/the-surprising-way-to-feel-less-busy.

[69] Zoë Chance, "How to make a behaviour addictive," *TEDxMillRiver* (May 14, 2013), https://www.youtube.com/watch?v=AHfiKav9fcQ.

[70] Carol Ewing Garber et al., "Quantity and Quality of Exercise for Developing and Maintaining Cardiorespiratory, Musculoskeletal, and Neuromotor Fitness in Apparently Healthy Adults: Guidance for Prescribing Exercise," *Medicine & Science in Sports & Exercise* 43, no. 7 (July 2011): 1334-1359, https://journals.lww.com/acsm-msse/Fulltext/2011/07000/Quantity_and_Quality_of_Exercise_for_Developing.26.aspx.

[71] Adam Sinicki, "The downsides of wearing a fitness tracker,"

(blog), September 7 (year not listed), accessed March 4, 2018, http://www.healthguidance.org/entry/17514/1/The-Downsides-o f-Wearing-a-Fitness-Tracker.html.

[72] Feedback from the first group that completed the challenge: They would have liked reminders throughout the day to complete the challenges; i.e., more nudges. So, in later groups, reminder emails were also sent out at 11:00 a.m. and 3:00 p.m.

[73] "More Grey Hair on Facebook As Baby Boomers Become Fastest Growing Social Media Demographic," Castleford (blog), April 18, 2016, https://www.castleford.com.au /content-marketing-blog/more-grey-hair-on-facebook-as-baby-bo omers-become-fastest-growing-social-media-demographic/.

[74] Data on trends in social media access by older adults was listed at the link below and accessed on March 6, 2018 (the research report has since been restricted to paid users only). https://www.smartinsights.com/social-media-marketing/social-media-strategy/new-global-social-media-research/.

[75] These facts were also shared with me by a social media consultant during a networking event in 2016.

[76] Yes, I'm dating myself with the reference to mixed tapes. Today, it would be a playlist on a music streaming service. But it still accomplishes the same thing.

[77] You can watch one of our VERY early obstacle courses on my YouTube channel. This one (https://youtu.be/qovAC_Yw_j0) was circa winter 2007—pre-social media savvy for me! The course was pretty basic; they actually got more elaborate and physically

demanding. And fun! I always completed the courses with my kids.

[78] David Halpern, *Inside the Nudge Unit: How Small Changes Can Make A Big Difference* (London: WH Allen, 2015).

[79] Halpern, *Inside the Nudge Unit.*

[80] Ingenium (website), accessed April 12, 2018, https://ingeniumcanada.org.

[81] "Barriers to Physical Activity," Centers for Disease Control and Prevention (website), accessed January 30, 2018, https://www.cdc.gov/physicalactivity/basics/adding-pa/barriers.html.

[82] As a personal trainer, I hear many of these excuses from current and potential clients. One of my roles as a trainer is to help people understand how they can overcome these barriers, so that they are not being held back by excuses and blockages.

[83] *2013/2014 Staying@Work Report, Canada Summary,* (Toronto: Willis Towers Watson, February 2014), https://www.towerswatson.com/en-CA/Insights/IC-Types/Survey-Research-Results/2014/02/2013-2014-staying-at-work-report-canada-summary.

FURTHER READING

Want to learn more? Check out some of these great authors:

Bowman, Katy. *Move Your DNA: Restore Your Health Through Natural Movement*. United States of America: Propriometrics Press, 2014.

Cuddy, Amy. *Presence: Bringing Your Boldest Self To Your Biggest Challenges*. New York: Little, Brown and Company, 2015.

Duhigg, Charles. *The Power of Habit—Why We Do What We Do in Life and Business*. New York: Random House, 2012.

Esmonde-White, Miranda. *Aging Backwards: 10 Years Younger, 10 Years Lighter, 30 Minutes a Day*. Toronto: Random House Canada, 2014.

Halpern, David. *Inside the Nudge Unit: How Small Changes Can Make A Big Difference*. London: WH Allen, 2015.

Levine, James A., and Selene Yeager. *Move a Little, Lose A Lot: New NEAT Science Reveals How to Be Thinner, Happier, and Smarter*. New York: Crown Publishing, 2009.

Vernikos, Joan. *Sitting Kills, Moving Heals: How Simple Everyday Movement Will Prevent Pain, Illness, and Early Death—and Exercise Alone Won't*. Fresno: Quill Driver Books, 2011.

Wiking, Meik. *The Little Book of Lykke: The Danish Search for the World's Happiest People*. Canada: Penguin Random House, 2017.

AUTHOR'S NOTE

Thank you so much to my wonderful family—Emily, Simon, and Tim—for supporting and encouraging every crazy, hare-brained scheme I have (and for talking me off the ledge when they are a little too hare-brained). Thank you to my parents—Mary and Alex—for being early guinea pigs in my fitness journey. Your unconditional love is forever appreciated.

Patrick Smith, your athleticism and unwavering commitment to your goals inspire me. I am grateful that you agreed to be interviewed for this book, and I thank you for taking time out of your busy training schedule.

Thanks to Sheri Burge, Jeanne Wright, and Cassandra McCoy for being friends without borders. Your support, kindness, and humour keep me sustained.

My stellar editorial team helped me create a fantastic book: Kaarina, Dianna, Matthew, and Jennifer. You made the journey of self-publishing rewarding and so much less scary. Fellow authors Kate Jaimet and Stacey Atkinson provided moral support and advice to a newbie author. Friends and family alike helped me choose the best cover for this book: Tim, Emily, Simon, Mary, Steph, Sheri, Jeanne, and Cassandra.

And last but not least, I owe a debt of gratitude to all of my fitness clients. You've put your bodies and well-being in my hands, and I appreciate your trust in my abilities as a fitness professional. Keep moving.

ABOUT THE AUTHOR

Amanda Sterczyk is an ACSM Certified Personal Trainer and a Certified Essentrics® Instructor. In 2016, she founded The Move More Institute™, an initiative to promote healthy active living by adding more exercise and non-exercise activity to individuals' daily lives.

Amanda Sterczyk Fitness offers in-home/in-office personal training, Essentrics® group/private sessions, and movement coaching/workshops in central Ottawa, Canada, and online, as well as online personal training via Skype/FaceTime/Zoom. Amanda specializes in helping retired older adults and sedentary office workers maintain strength, flexibility, and mobility. She has been teaching group fitness classes since 2010. Amanda has taught men, women, and children of all ages and ability levels, including elite athletes. Her slogan is: Move more, feel better.

Amanda holds a Master's degree in social psychology from Carleton University (1993). Before her career in fitness, she worked for over 10 years in health-promotion research and human resources.

She lives in Ottawa, Canada, with her husband, two teenage children, two gerbils, and one very clingy cat.

You can connect with Amanda online by visiting the following links:

http://www.amandasterczyk.com
https://www.facebook.com/AmandaSterczykFitness/
https://www.youtube.com/c/AmandaSterczykFitness
https://twitter.com/amanda_stretch
https://www.instagram.com/amanda_stretch/

Made in the USA
San Bernardino, CA
31 May 2019